THE DAMN DETOX

How Reconnecting to Yourself, is the Key to Health

by Amanda Gabbert

Certified Health Coach, Personal Trainer
and Energy Healer

ISBN# 978-1-7329958-3-3

Book design: Diana Wade
Cover photo: Say Cheese CLT, Mohammad Waheed
Back cover photo: Jcon Shots Photography, Julia Conway

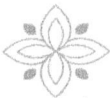

www.amanda-gabbert.com
Charlotte, North Carolina

TABLE OF CONTENTS

INTRODUCTION

Why call it The Damn Detox? The name of the book is not to deter you from the idea of detoxification, but rather to reflect that hopefully my own experience of it can offer you knowledge to improve your own detox.

Sometimes it takes an extreme situation, along with some mishaps, to recognize both the benefits and proper process which could be applied to the lives of others. I went through an intense bout of toxicity that was taxing on my mind, body and my soul. It started with a liver detox where I didn't fully understand what I was doing, and then a lot of other possible toxins that came out of the woodwork. Habits from the past, due to poor diet and medications, resurfaced simultaneously. You could say it was a perfect storm. My health crisis brought attention to the other areas of my life that needed improvement, especially the relationship I had with myself. Since this series of disasters and learning from them, I've become a Certified Health Coach, Personal Trainer and Energy Healer with my specialty in assisting clients in detox practices. Due to my own learnings, we add cleansing methods slowly but surely, to purify the mind and body. It's customized according to personal lifestyle and budget, so the client's quality of life is not hindered in the same severe way.

Why does detox often get a bad rap? Is it because it's bringing something to our attention that we need to do, but are resistant to? Often times we think of the word 'detox' in relation to a juice cleanse, water fast or something else that could be thought of as severe. I have fallen into this thought process as well, but by seeing how incredible this was and how small applications could prevent this feeling of restriction, it's my belief we can create more sustainable practices with small habits mentally, physically and spiritually. Yes, the body can detox on its own, however the problem is the burden we place on it in a standard day. With most energy focused on digestion, you can only imagine how little gets directed to detox. Especially in times of emotional stress, sickness and with the hundreds of other responsibilities the body has chemically, supporting detox is not just an option in my opinion, it's a way of living for longevity, energy and quality of life. Allowing toxic build-up is inevitable over time, and the amount of toxins in our environment are also growing.

In today's world, the word 'toxin' has a multitude of meanings. Whether it be in our water, chemicals in our prescription medications, or heavy metals in our vaccinations. Even the air we breathe can pull in toxins from the pollution of fuels and the increase in manufacturers due to our demands on the material world. Alongside, the physical world, emotions can also become congested in the body and express themselves as physical ailments or aches and pains. All of these toxins gradually accumulate over time and inhibit our body from doing what it does best, which is regenerating cells for healing, absorbing nutrients from our food, carrying oxygen through our blood, creating and assimilating hormones, and so much more. Too many toxins can even prevent us from properly eliminating them when it becomes physically overwhelming. But I don't want you to live life in fear of everything we encounter. Just like everything else, there's a proper balance in awareness as to what is entering our bodies, and how we can effectively help ourselves through detoxification.

There are many different types of detoxing, whether it's a full body detox with a variety of supplementation, or something like a juice cleanse with the purpose of giving your digestive tract a break. Although the liver gallbladder flush created some heavy disturbances in my own body, understanding the importance of consistency, this form of detox was pivotal for me. Water fasting, intermittent fasting and many other fasts are also increasing in popularity. We all eat differently and have different lifestyles, so how we detox is going to be unique to each and every one of us. We are all comprised of a different history that has conditioned us, different foods we grew up on and different genetic backgrounds. Who's to tell us that we should all be doing the same kind of detoxification? Anything we intentionally put in our body is our decision, and in turn we have some additional decisions as to what and how we take things out.

The process of detoxification is much more than removing chemical toxins from your body. These chemical toxins can also prevent you from thinking clearly and being at your happiest due to the inhibition of brain biochemicals and neurotransmitters, hormones and many other collaborative functions in the body. Through my detox process, I experienced everything from ADHD to anxiety, from depression to brain fog. I had to learn to separate my body from my personality and spirit, so I could continue to be motivated and happy in my life to get through this process. It was a difficult task to continue striving forward some days, however if I had not recognized the physical effects of these toxins and remembered the person I knew I was, I would have allowed them to take over mentally, preventing my drive to continue healing and living my life. Acceptance as to where we are in life, can create inner peace and support desired results.

Years of unprocessed emotions and beliefs were part of this detoxification as well. In learning more about past events that I was still holding on to, I came to realize some of these emotions were contributing to health issues I had in the past as well as presently. The beautiful thing about this however, is although it was challenging to both physically and emotionally detox at the same time, I got a two-for-one deal and the ability to start fresh in many facets. Sometimes we hold on to pain we have experienced in the past caused by other people, whether it be judgment for our body types, being made fun of on the playground in school, or maybe some of that emotional abuse from previous relationships that created feelings of worthlessness. Although these contribute to our hurt in the past, the fact that we continue to hold on to past trauma only ends up affecting our current and future relationships, and outward actions and reactions. We begin to project our pain and dissatisfaction onto others, creating a ripple effect of negativity and hurt. Giving ourselves permission to let go of all of this through forgiveness and self-acceptance can go hand-in-hand with the health of our bodies. This allows us to move forward with a life full of happiness and joy-both energies that we can feel more pleased of in gifting to those around us.

During my toxicity, I had to learn what it meant to advocate for myself. A big component to my detoxification was listening to my body and giving it what it needed. Only you can have an intuitive sense about what your body physically and chemically requires, and this becomes more prevalent during the detoxification process as we open pathways that were once blocked. Of course, having a physician to guide us along our path and proper testing to confirm or disprove theories can be essential, but at the end of the day, we know our bodies best and we must be able to tap into these responses, so we can act as our own cheerleader. Being capable of communicating our thoughts and emotions effectively to providers can not only provide us with the confidence we need in the world of health, but translate to healthier relationships outside of the doctor's office.

If I hadn't taken the time to look up the details on my blood-work, different kinds of supplementation and alternate therapies, I'm not sure what my condition would be right now. This is not to insinuate that you cannot trust leaders in the medical world, it means that we need to team up and work together, preparing ourselves to ask questions so that everyone involved can be their best self. We have the ability to decide for ourselves what our health is worth to us, and how long we want to be on this planet. Sure, we cannot see the future and what our timeline looks like. Regardless of our fated paths free will is always a variable. However, if we are living in the present to consider the future, releasing anything that no longer serves us on all levels can allow us to co-create our realities.

Throughout this book I share with you my personal story on detoxification along with advice that I integrate in my coaching program. You will notice in the back of the book additional pages are provided. I did this for two reasons: 1) To make it seem like I wrote a lot more than I did (the jokes come free), and 2) because I want this experience to be interactive and provide you a place to take notes. If you have a whole lot bubbling up while you read and reflect, you might want to grab an additional notebook. Maybe that will be the beginning of your own published story, like it was mine.

Let's get you back to who you want to be and what you desire. Whether it be attempting a half marathon, feeling more excited about life, or skipping down the block with your grandkids, we all deserve exactly what we want when it comes to health and wellness, and we can become more aware and empowered to make this happen for ourselves with the right support. I hope my story can inspire you to live a fulfilling life of love for yourself and others.

Chapter 1: My Damn Detox

*M*y head feels like it's going to explode, I have an unnerving sensation all over my body, and just the idea of someone or something brushing against me makes me want to shoot through the roof. I haven't had a period in a few months, my muscles feel so tight and stiff that working out is not an option. My once flawless complexion is now ravaged with acne. I'm exhausted and can't eat enough avocado toast to save my life. My life took a huge change in the spring of 2017 and it seemed impossible at the time to figure out what was the cause of all of this, no matter how many doctors were involved. I decided I would have to put together my own story as to where this might be coming from, recalling previous life events and how that might have contributed in accumulating to show these symptoms. Typically, I claim every New Year how I will dominate the next 12 months, but it seemed the universe had another plan in mind.

In the fall of 2016, about 6 months early, I had been experiencing symptoms of indigestion, fatigue, sleeplessness, and nausea, with no clue as to why. I had been attempting to change my habits by reading about natural remedies and how certain foods can support the body. I took the opportunity to try different diets as I went through a Health Coaching program, seeing as my interest in health and well-being had sparked even further. This also allowed me to experiment in case I might recommend certain eating tactics to future clients. In my many attempts to improve these symptoms, it seemed no matter what I ate or how much I eliminated from my diet proved successful. This began to heighten my concern. None of what was happening to me in my current state was making much sense, so I began to piece it together as I reviewed my past even further.

I'd kept developing sinus infections back to back after moving to Charlotte, North Carolina from St. Louis, Missouri in 2014. With a history of outdoor allergies, I knew I was being exposed to a different variety with my regional change in residence. With these consistent respiratory problems, I was being prescribed a different antibiotic monthly for about seven consecutive months. I was thinking, 'What could possibly be wrong with me?!' It was eventually recommended I take an allergy test and although I did have some expected outdoor allergies, wheat came up as an offender in foods. It initiated a change in thought for me when it comes to how we support our bodies with nutrition. I always knew I wanted to be healthy and eat healthy, but sometimes the understanding of what is in our minds may not be the same definition our physical body agrees with. Wheat is nutritious and high in protein, but for my own personal chemistry it was a threat and consuming it meant I experienced constipation, indigestion and sinus infections. As a result, some damage had been done to my digestive tract, and I knew it was going to take time to repair. I was incredibly relieved however after seeing fewer sinus infections and less digestive distress from simply eliminating a food. Eureka!

I did occasionally have a "cheat meal" with wheat and realized that after its elimination, my body was having an even harder time digesting it. I concluded that the pain was no longer worth the splurges and cut it out entirely. So long to the incredibly tempting warm pretzels during hockey games. Goodbye to the Thanksgiving rolls, stuffing and pie - I will miss you, but you're killing me.

I'd felt amazing for the couple of years following this food elimination and lost fifteen pounds! It was time to start looking at the chemistry of what was occurring inside my body, versus what the mirror was reflecting. Although my new-found gluten-free life was treating me well and I considered myself even healthier, I was still sure to make up for lost cravings on the weekends with other goodies. I would order my gluten-free pizza and go out with my friends in the evenings, slamming vodkas with club soda, because, you know, they're only 80 calories each and weekly stress wasn't going to cure itself! So, a portion of my perspective was still skewed when it came to health, yet I was on a slow but sure journey of learning what a holistic and natural life meant for me.

I had been taking an anti-depressant, Duloxetine, as well as birth control in the form of oral contraceptives. These both started at about the age of 18. Because if a girl's hormones aren't to blame for her mood swings as a teenager, let's just put her on an additional medication. Ironically, as I cut out wheat, my depression cleared itself. I decided to slowly go off the Duloxetine as I felt it wasn't necessary anymore. Unfortunately, I fainted shortly after...a couple of times. Once when I was on a date, and another time when I was out with friends in the evening. Damage had been done to my vagus nerve effecting blood flow, creating what was labeled as a vasovagal syncope (if you're not familiar, the vagus nerve is a pretty big portion of the central nervous system, coming from the brain and connecting to most of your organs sending them energy to function). When I went to my doctor, they simply had no solution or understanding as to why these happened. After doing my own digging, I feel the long-term use of Duloxetine could have been the cause. Serotonin is affected by the vagus nerve since many organs including the gut, are controlled by that nerve. Most serotonin is produced in the gut and outside of the digestive issues, Duloxetine (also called Cymbalta) has been linked to serotonin syndrome.[1] This is the bio-chemical responsible for keeping us relaxed throughout the day and easing us into sleep at night. Unfortunately, many drugs often cause more damage for the same symptoms they are indicated to fix because the body gets used to their say so and adjusts. Then, when you come off of them, the body has to get reacclimated and that can take quite a long time depending on how long you have been taking a medication. In order to get sleep, I took the supplements melatonin and another version of tryptophan called 5-HTP, which converts more readily to serotonin. Bedtime tea with some powdered magnesium citrate were also staples of my nighttime routine.

The birth control changed my chemistry over time, too. As women we do whatever we can to take precaution if children are not planned for our near future, so we medicate to change the biological functions of our body's natural cycle. After about eight years of a particular birth control, I went to my doctor and explained I didn't feel it was working anymore. I had issues with spotting and I wasn't sure why. She said there shouldn't be an issue, but we could try another one. Again, of all the technology we have, there was no testing to discover hormone levels and if there could be a problem? I trusted that my best interest was being taken into consideration and tried a couple of different forms of birth control after our conversation. One made me feel incredibly anxious and moody, so I switched REAL quick.

The next birth control caused a flood of estrogen in my body, leading to melasma. Melasma is hormonal pigmentation that comes to the surface of the skin. Essentially, I looked like I had a light mustache as well as two giant spots on my cheeks and one between my eyebrows. Oh, how the single-life confidence took a step back on this one!

Eventually, I decided to go for the most natural route promoted, which I understood would get me off added hormones. I chose the Paragard IUD (Intrauterine Device). I hated the idea of something floating for up to 10 years in my body, but I was tired of feeling as if I was being pumped full of estrogen. It seemed to work pretty well right out of the gate. My cycles took some time to regulate, but I was also cycling every three months on the previous medication, so I assumed that would be the case. I noticed as my hormones normalized to what my body needed, I had new hair growth! Who knew birth control could change that quality?! Look out Pantene, a new model is headed your direction! Once I noticed this, I thought, "What else could have been effected by my hormones?"

I came across a few articles on oral contraceptives and their relationship to gallstones. Did you know that these preventative medications can cause bile to back up into the gallbladder and then form stones?[2] Indigestion is a sign of low stomach acid or bile, not too much. If stones hinder bile production, this can prevent the breakdown of your food and allow bad bacteria to overgrow in the intestinal tract, as bile is a natural way to keep this balance. How many women can you think of in your life that are missing a gallbladder? Could this be why?

As I continued to read about the relationship of the gallbladder and the liver, I realized I had a lot of signs that indicated some congestion in the liver. The indigestion, a form of dermatitis around my mouth, and developing a productive cough after I ate, seemed to consistently relate back to the liver in my research. It's amazing how some symptoms just become so normal in our lives that we don't realize that they are in fact indicators that something is happening. I even had high iron and liver enzymes on my physicals the past two years, and what did the doctor say when I asked? "It's nothing to be concerned about." Let me say here that when numbers are in red on your lab work, it's something to be concerned about. Your liver is responsible for over 500 biochemical processes, so one problem in that department can indicate potential issues throughout the rest of the body.[3]

During the course work for my Health Coaching certification, videos would pop-up with similar facts and information that I was reading on my own about liver health. Sometimes the world will lead us to the answers we are searching for, so remain open and pay attention to acknowledge what you are being presented. One video I watched was a presentation by an ayurvedic doctor and he brought up a liver/gallbladder flush. This is a way to detox the body and safely soften and release any stones that could be accumulating in the gallbladder and liver (there are such a thing as liver stones as well, but they typically don't show up in scans, hence their lack of acknowledgment). I found a video on a liver/gallbladder flush by a doctor who was mentioned in the past by a friend from the gym. More synchronicity! I looked at the protocol and although intense, I was already cutting so many foods out and playing with all the different diets I was learning, that a strict vegetarian regimen with light snacking, tons of apple cider vinegar and herbs was a challenge I was ready to take on.

It was prescribed that after five days of these dietary changes, the sixth day calls for fasting, drinking a measured amount of Epsom salts mixed with water a couple of times a day, as well as a lemon and olive oil mixture right before bed. Epsom salts open your bile duct so the stones you have softened can pass through gently, as your body is stimulated to secrete bile by the fats in the olive oil. The next day, or the "flush" day, you will literally be doing such... all day long (you're welcome). Stones will continue to pass through your gallbladder and liver, allowing them to eventually function at a higher capacity. If this is something that interests you, I'm giving you the shortened version and I also urge you to speak with a health professional first, as I learned the hard way that there are downsides to jumping into extreme detoxification with little supervision. Consistency is key with this protocol as well, repeating it monthly until you see no stones.

The night after my flush day I experienced an insomnia I never knew existed. I was scared that something was seriously wrong with me as I stared at my phone in the wee hour of 2:00am. I obviously wouldn't be sleeping in the near future, so I emailed the supplement company I purchased the cleanse protocol from to be sure there was nothing I should be concerned about. To my surprise, they answered quickly, and explained about what's called the Herxheimer Reaction. This is a physical response your body can have due to the overwhelming amount of toxins you release in the detoxification process. If your body cannot process them quickly enough, (which depends on the individual and their history of toxins), they can cause other symptoms. For me, it was insomnia, but for someone else it could make them feel flu-like, disoriented, or tired. Anything could result, depending on how your body responds to toxins or typically displays side effects. If you release so much that your body cannot get rid of everything at once, it will reaccumulate in other tissues. I got about two hours of forced sleep thanks to a magnesium supplement, until the alarm pierced through the dark at 6am to fly to New York the next day for a Christmas weekend of fun.

What do you do in New York when you visit for only two nights? You drink coffee, eat 'til you're nearly sick, and drink, drink, drink! And I'm not referring to water. Unfortunately, given that I'd just detoxed, this was the worst thing I could have possibly done. Not understanding at that time how many toxins were in my body, or how to properly give the body space to remove them, my body took all the energy that remained and refocused its attention on digestion. I didn't want to inhibit anyone else's New York experience, even though all I truly wanted was rest. Digestion by itself takes up a significant amount our body's energy. If we get sick, this is a big reason why getting that extra downtime and sipping on broth helps us recover quickly. Our digestive tract is the first pathway in detoxification, and in my case it was preoccupied with coffee, food, and more toxins in the form of alcohol, while all that I released went elsewhere.

Those circulating toxins took up home in my blood stream, lymph system, and fatty tissues. All those years of medications, a diet of processed foods in my earlier years, and previously drowned emotions that had nowhere to go, mixed with the enormous amounts of alcohol that I had attempted to wash them away with, were all released at once. They consumed me, and I unknowingly allowed it. Self-sabotage much?

As the next couple months went by, I noticed I would have a day here and there where I ironically felt the word best to describe it was "toxic." I would feel unusually tired, weak and foggy. Still not realizing that's what it was, I continued to go along in my merry life, thinking I had done something extraordinary for myself and was taking back my health in my own hands. I did do something great for myself in the long run, but the uphill hike was exhausting. I initiated myself on the hamster wheel of two-year detox.

Now we're back to the current state of my health first described. Symptoms started to grow, and sickness was overcoming my body. I couldn't sleep, felt miserable, had terrible headaches as if my brain was literally punching my skull. Tight muscles, horrible fatigue, and my nerves were so tender and sensitive I wanted to crawl into a ball and be left alone. I was craving starches and fats so badly, along with sodium. My skin started breaking out severely and I could feel the urgency to go to the bathroom was infrequent. I knew this meant there was something wrong with my urinary tract, and on top of it I was three months late for a period. Although the previous paragraphs seem simple enough to piece my story together, I was not quite convinced as to the cause in this moment. I visited three doctors and no one was sure as to what was going on. I was terrified many nights as to whether or not I would wake up the next morning. I'd lay in bed crying, feeling hopeless, alone, and confused. I knew I would do whatever it took, but I had no clue as to what that was.

I never thought life would throw an experience like this my way. I was young, smart, motivated, and had a good heart. I was one of the healthiest eaters of the people I knew, and I exercised all the time. Was this not the route to success? Sometimes we do not realize how much fight we have in us until our life depends on it. I had to change my perspective quickly, understanding that this was not a punishment, but a catalyst to get me to the future I so desired. I put on my gloves, stepped into the ring, and said, "Bring it on. I will not stop until I have answers."

Synchronicity popped up again when I met my current naturopath at a farmer's market. According to the sign in front of her cash register, she was a doctor in addition to selling organic herbs, and specialized in detoxification. I knew she was in my path for a reason. I had not been very spiritual in the past few years, although I still believed in a higher power, so you better believe I started praying my ass off. I was constantly asking for guidance and strength to get me through. Sometimes divine timing and our time are not one in the same, but ask and you shall receive—maybe even a doctor vending at a market. I spoke briefly with the Naturopath on my situation and in just a few minutes, she spouted off more solutions and test options for me than all three of the previous doctors combined. She had me at "hello."

Finally feeling as if I was being heard, a couple weeks later

I saw her at my initial appointment. She asked what my health had been like since the very beginning. Not the beginning of the year prior—she meant since birth. It's often overlooked how important this is. I was born via C-section, which does not expose babies to the natural bacteria they would encounter passing through a mother's vaginal tract. These bacteria help build the immune system.[4] Immediately following birth, I contracted a life-threatening version of staph in the hospital. Life was off to a rough start. Years of antibiotics in my youth and early adulthood killed the good bacteria in my body as well as the bad, and of course the most recent happenings all gave insight as to what the condition of my body was currently.

When asked about my latest form of birth control, she warned me that the Paragard IUD could cause copper allergy or copper toxicity. Sometimes very few signs are associated with this and it can be fatal if it goes on too long before being identified.[5] So, we went forward with a heavy metals test and when the results came in, it showed my zinc was extremely high but copper was normal. Too much copper can displace your zinc however, so I thought I finally had my answer! I immediately called my OBGYN and explained the situation. They wouldn't be able to get me in for a few days and they were not willing to budge. I wanted this thing out immediately and was in no mood to wait. I even called them back to ask if they had reported the device as doctors should if there is an adverse event (any occurrence that could indicate it contributed to death or serious injury or illness).[6] The nurse's explanation was simply, "Well you're the first we've ever heard this from." So no, the answer was they didn't care to fulfill their duties and avoided reporting information that could have potentially saved other lives. Luckily, I had established myself with a functional medicine doctor who was also an OBGYN, and when I called they got me in immediately. That IUD was out in no time. Good riddance!

I still had many other tests run to check gut bacteria, analyze by-products that could be causing harmful chemical output, along with a general blood test to get an overall picture. I did tons of alternate therapies- cryotherapy, IV therapy, reiki, infrared sauna and the list goes on- as they supported me in trying to keep active to maintain my health in another way, and of course I also needed to keep my day job to afford my natural healing route. The bacteria in my gut, or microbiome as it's commonly referred to, were out of whack as the toxins I was eliminating were feeding negative strains on their way out. It was constantly a catch 22, so the more I detoxed, the more I had to watch my diet and be leery of possible tummy side effects. I even did some genetic testing that allowed me to find out I had a mutation when it came to my liver detox pathway, and I now had to cut out heavily sulfur-based foods. This includes cruciferous vegetables like kale, brussel sprouts, broccoli, cauliflower, onion, and garlic. So, although I was trying to eat healthy, it was difficult when many vegetables were not personally good for me, and I had to watch sugars from fruits. When your body is in a heightened immune state, if you eat the same thing consistently, it can begin to see it as a threat, so I was juggling foods as much as I could with my minimized choices.

As time went on, I realized the pain in under my right rib was accumulating and I felt a ton of pressure pushing against it. Yellowing of the eyes slowly showed itself and that was my cue…

it was my liver. Jaundice is something we typically associate with yellow eyes and poor liver function. This guy (yes, I talk to my liver now) had been through so much in trying to process all these toxins. For the next year and a half, I did liver flush, after flush, using a similar protocol mentioned in the first one I completed. This cleanse however included apple juice or malic acid to soften stones, along with Epsom salts in water and olive oil. I would do one about every 3 weeks, however if I felt the pressure accumulate again earlier than that, I went for it. Towards the end of this 'healthscapade', I did one weekly for six consecutive weeks to speed up the process. After reading more on the subject on liver flushing, it is recommended that you conduct a flush every month after the first one until you see no stones for two flushes in a row.

There was emotional work to do as well as the physical. I parted from relationships along the way, which brought attention to the personality types I was surrounding myself with. Reflecting on my nurturing nature, and always keeping quiet on how I felt to please others, I realized this in and of itself could be the reason I was sick. I gave all my energy away and did not know who I was. In having to remain focused on my health while learning to let people and personal habits go, I've realized if we have a healthy perspective on life, speak our truth and love ourselves, everything else including physical health habits will follow. Energy is part of an exchange on all levels, so giving without receiving can very well drain us.

Do you believe you deserve the healthiest version of you? What is your reasoning for wanting this in the first place? If we don't understand why we are wanting something in our lives, we are bound to fail. Intentions and mindset allow us to define our version of success. If you truly want to do something for yourself, there's got to be a 'why' to support it. It could be as simple as "I want to lose weight, so I can live a longer happier life" to as extreme as "I've always dreamed of climbing Mt. Everest." Whatever reason or reasons pop into your head immediately, write them down. Close your eyes and envision yourself in the future, feeling free of minor aches and pains, digestive issues, etc. What sensations come over your body? How exciting does it feel to be that person you want to be? Sometimes allowing ourselves even the opportunity to imagine what a balanced life can bring, is enough motivation in itself.

Therefore, the first step in detoxing is WANTING it. Health is not a trend, it's a lifestyle. So many people desire to be healthy, however once they realize the consistency and thought that must go into it, they back away. This happens to all of us in some way shape or form, and some of us have more difficulty than others. Many of us must go through something drastic to really take things to the next level. Ask yourself, how bad are you willing to let your health get before you make changes? Are you one of the lucky ones and started early, or are you later in life and find yourself with multiple metabolic issues causing chronic ailments? Wherever you find yourself, there are ways you can ease into detoxification. And the best part is, if you start slowly and take one bite out of the paleo pie at a time, you won't have to encounter an extreme incident to wake you up.

When it comes to health, the most important relationship is the one we have with ourselves. We tend to compare ourselves to others, rather than looking inward and being grateful for what we have and who we are. Comparison is the result of fear distracting us from bettering ourselves and facing our emotions head on. It's my hope that not only will you begin to desire a physically active and nutritionally abundant life as you read this book, but you understand how relationships with others, the world and yourself equally contribute to your sense of well-being. Our bodies were born knowing its needs on a biochemical and intuitive level, and in reconnecting with it, we can redesign our life to fulfill our dreams. This allows us to hand the reins over to our body, creating a trusting relationship physically, emotionally and energetically. Let go and flow.

Detoxification is something that everyone should consider, however there are extreme experiences where education and guidance can be supportive. Understanding how dedicated and consistent detoxification should be is essential, but there are also ways we can easily incorporate small but sure habits. As we move forward, I will give you some tips and tricks in learning how to detoxify your life, so you can feel more in tune with your body, happier, healthier and more purposeful in your everyday.

In the following chapters, I will discuss what I recommend to clients and friends, while asking some thought-provoking questions. Read on to better understand my path, what actions might best apply to your life, and how health coaching and energy healing could benefit in supporting your potential lifestyle changes. Let's do The Damn Detox.

Chapter 2: Check Yourself, Before You Wreck Yourself

*O*ften times in life we have a tendency to see the cup half empty. With negativity all around us, it can be very easy to fall into this gap and be unaware that it's even happening. It can also depend on your personality type, along with your awareness and the types of environments you are putting yourself in. Do you have more leadership qualities versus following the crowd? Are you empathic and sensitive? Do you give more than you receive? Do you know how to receive or feel deserving of what your heart would like to see in this lifetime? I sure didn't!

Going back to that beautiful intuition, learning to resonate with the feeling on where we are in life in at any given moment can guide us to what we would like to result and our ultimate purpose. What do you think your purpose is on this earth? Is it enough for you or do you hope to do more? Are you being who you want to be, or what others prefer you to be? What changes would you like to make on how you perceive yourself and the world around you? The best part is we can always decide to take action and evolve who we are into who we would feel more fulfilled in being.

MY DETOX
My perspective on life used to be as pessimistic and paranoid

as it could get. I always thought of myself as a victim, looking at what people were doing to me, versus understanding why I was attracting the personalities I had. I was incredibly hard on myself, and thought nothing I ever did was good enough. I had multiple failed romantic relationships with men, and always seemed to find the narcissist of the bunch. In my case, and for so many others, it can seem as if once you date one, they all can smell you from a mile away. Getting constantly verbally knocked down not only lowered my self-esteem, but confirmed my inward belief that I was "not good enough." It becomes cyclical, and no matter how much pain is experienced, when we are acquainted with a particular feeling (good or bad) there is a level of safety in it and a great fear in walking away from that comfort.

In 2015, I went through a devastating break-up. I think in the back of my head I knew I deserved so much better, and of course wanted better, but it was a small bud that was on its way to flowering as I remained in my unsafe but safe zone. When he left, I was traumatized. My inner victim kept the internal dialogue going of "why does this keep happening to me?" and "how come I never receive the love I give?" As this had happened multiple times before, I decided to talk myself out of the fetal position. Why was I constantly allowing other people to have such an emotional effect on my life? I was always doing for others and never enough for myself, and then resented them and their lack of support. So not only was I setting myself up to feel less than by staying in these relationships, I projected the same feeling of unworthiness I had for myself on others. Friends and family then also never felt good enough when they were with me.

I never intended to make anyone feel this way, however

sometimes when we internalize feelings about ourselves, we see others through the same lens and indirectly allow them to feel our pain. There's a quote from an unknown source I always think of now to help me through any situation: "Your perception of me is a reflection of you; my reaction to you is an awareness of me." Any time we are about to judge a person or a situation, it helps to realize that whatever their response may be, good or bad, reflects their life experience and how they see themselves. At the same time, how we perceive someone is a mirror of emotions we have toward ourselves. So now if I see someone and I begin to judge them, I ask myself, "How is this a reflection of something I am unhappy with on the inside? What belief about myself do I need to heal?"

As an example of this quote, through my most recent physical healing process, my acne was such an embarrassment to me. I had to constantly remind myself that my soul and body are two different things, and I should be grateful to my physical body for everything it's persevered through, rather than critiquing it. One day, someone said to me, "[anonymous] told me your skin never used to look like that," and it absolutely broke my heart. In one regard, it made me feel as if I was being talked about behind my back, but I was also already ruminating on it myself. As I talked with her about my health journey, I realized she had insecurities in her own skin and the pain I felt from her comment was the pain she was holding in herself. In discussing the situation with her, my vulnerability gave her permission to open-up as well. She probably needed someone to relate to, which is most likely why we were in each other's paths. I had empathy for her and that allowed me to let go of the hurt feelings, realizing what I felt was simply a transfer of her own emotions, having nothing to do with me personally. It also forced me to recognize the depth of my own self-criticism and what I needed to let go of in focusing on my appearance.

The only person that needed to love me at the end of the day was me. I had avoided caring about my wants and needs for so long because to an extent, caring for others and seeing them smile is what makes me happy. There's a balance to this though, and the understanding that many people can spot this nurturing side and take advantage of it if they have not been nurtured otherwise. But 'taking advantage', is actually us allowing it simultaneously. They may not even know it sometimes, but many of us desire love, and at some point in our lives we have not received the love we craved. Occasionally, we then come across those people so willing to smother us in it and it feels good. I don't blame anyone who allowed themselves to enjoy it, because I can understand where they are coming from, and part of me still loved giving it. I love some love too, and I am grateful to experiences of my past for showing me what I needed to learn in order to find a better nurturing balance.

Have you ever heard someone say that we are a result of the five people we hang out with the most? A friend mentioned this to me a few years ago and in my head, I immediately said, "Oh shit." There were a few people I was socializing with regularly I knew were not a great influence on me, and they mimicked some of the qualities of my romantic relationships. I gave, and they received. I felt guilty if I didn't and they would do what they could to confirm my fears of not being good enough. That was about it. Their insecurities ruled their life and they lived it in fear, but at the same time that's how I operated, which is why I attracted it. Their fears became my fears and vice versa, due to those pesky projections again. I lived a stagnant life in a box, versus thinking of all the opportunities I could make available to myself because this fear created impenetrable hypothetical walls.

After feeling I had lost who I was in my relationships, the first struggle in self-love, was not even knowing where to begin. I read a ton of self-development books to understand the perspectives on personal growth and relationships, and this action in itself was empowering me daily. This has become a consistent habit in my life as I feel motivated in listening to other strong writers, podcasters, etc., discussing subjects on self-improvement, self-love and living life in a healthy more passionate way. Sometimes even when we feel alone in our process, knowing other people like us exist is comforting, even via a pair of headphones.

Along the way, I noticed this more positive, motivated perspective was forcing negative influencers out of my life and drawing more like-minded individuals in. I had heard of the Law of Attraction, and something way back from that physics class notebook full of stars and hearts- the Law of Conservation of Energy. "Energy is neither created nor destroyed" so it will always exist, even if it takes a different form or transfers from one energy conductor to another. I had never imagined that an energetic exchange happened from person to person until I began to see it occur in my own life. Often a skeptic and being born in the "Show Me" state, I always needed proof that applied to my own experience before I'd be convinced. As I saw the changes around me, I began to open myself up more to the understanding that I was capable of drawing in healthier relationships, and they flowed freely to me. When we raise our energetic vibration, we attract like energies. Sometimes faith in the abstract is necessary for the beginning of a ripple effect.

In reflecting on who I wanted to be for my future happiness, I looked back to my early college years and wondered where that spunky ball of sass had disappeared to. I had known what I wanted, and I wasn't afraid to say it or do it. Granted at that age there were also sometimes I probably should have kept my mouth shut, there were still a lot of characteristics I wanted to return. Looking at how I interpreted hurt in the past and the pain I was still holding on to, I understood there were a lot of moments that I blamed other people for my lack of accomplishments in life. Rather, I should have been taking responsibility for my role in the decisions that got me there to begin with. In conjunction with this, I was holding onto a lot of anger and resentment. There's a theory that we hold specific emotions in different internal organs. Can you guess where anger and resentment reside? The liver and gallbladder.

Let the forgiveness commence! I don't know that I ever realized how much certain events effected my life, and how much emotion I was holding on to until I decided to dig deeper into it. This applies to us all. There will always be those moments that we do something, and it clicks in our brain as to where that response, emotion or habit came from. This could be good or bad, but when it comes to the bad and whoever is related to that, take a moment to reflect. Forgiveness for me was not an easy idea to wrap my head around, but when I realized how much this pain was controlling my life and I was giving away my power to these emotions, I was willing to forgive in a moment's notice to regain the person I knew.

The next step in my venture was connecting with what I loved to do in my free time. I had become so accustomed to my daily routine: going to the gym, to work, taking the dog for a walk, eating and prepping for the following day. Wow! "What a life," said sarcasm. I had lost sight if these things I did were even enjoyable to me, when I had so often followed along with what others did. "What did you love as a kid?" I read in one of my many encouraging books. This struck me. That kid was way cool, and I want to do what she did. I LOVED sports of any kind, and although I had been in recreational leagues as an adult in the past, I stopped. This was one of the many losses I was responsible for, always agreeing to what my friends or boyfriends wanted to do.

I started playing volleyball again, and I not only lifted weights as usual, I also started going to yoga more. I loved the strength and grace of it. I went to a dance class on occasion and incorporated aerial arts, too (you know the people that hang from fabric on the ceiling? That's the one.). I have always loved being creative, whether it be simply singing in the shower, painting, or sewing. Even giving myself a budget to redecorate on occasion. I felt so rejuvenated doing these things and began to incorporate them in my schedule on the reg. My inner child was beginning her healing.

YOUR DETOX

How do you perceive your life? What words come to mind? Health in this facet can go deep and many unknowns can come up. Behind our mindset is our perspective on life, and this can create habits we get locked into repeating. Do the people around you reflect who you are and who you want to be? What do you enjoy about your relationships? What do you dislike? What do you see in them that shows you something about yourself that could use improving?

Turn it Around
We have a responsibility when it comes to creating our own reality. We may not be able to dictate how others treat us, but we are the chief of our actions and reactions. If we perceive others are doing things "to us" rather than assume responsibility for why we think that way to begin with, we allow our lives to be ruined by others. Don't hate...co-create. How are these situations happening 'for us'? Turn it around.

Blaming ourselves for personal situations isn't necessary, as we all come from different backgrounds with different conditioning. Everyone involved, regardless as to the type of relationship, can take responsibility for their actions to one another, but beating ourselves up about the past only distracts us from moving forward. Forgiving others through understanding is important in releasing any heavy negative emotions we carry. Transferring one negative emotion to another, such as blame, is counterproductive to our goal.

There's a surge of energy that resides in our emotions, and they need to be released before it effects the physical body. None of us are going to be identical in thought, but to thrive as a community we should take the time to understand why people have the opinions they do. We may not agree with them or hope to get stuck in the "Big Brother" house together, but we can have compassion, and decide whether the relationship supports us in who we are and who we hope to be. If it doesn't, send them love anyway for their personal journey, and decide the boundaries of the relationship if it should continue at all. Having expectations of others can get us in trouble, because the stories we tell ourselves are not the stories that play out. Even if we're lucky and the end result is what we wanted, how we get places in life may look differently than the process we imagined. And sometimes that's a good thing!

No Expectations
Expectations come from fear and insecurity. No one is perfect nor will ever be completely rid of these pesky humanly characteristics. What we can do is be aware of these traits and catch them as they creep up, understanding how they could be affecting any decision making. Essentially, this life we lead has no walls. We create them as we don't know any better in our youth while attempting to fit in and abide by the "rules" others believe should apply. We do have control though in breaking these walls down as an adult. Then we can rebuild or edit the life we want most. This editing process can happen many times throughout our lives as things will always continue to change with growth. See gratitude in each moment rather than romanticizing what you lack, and release the expectations of yourselves and others. Visualize the feelings you would like to experience moment to moment or year to year and leave the expectations on how to get there or who will be a part of the process up to the Universe.

A Whole New World

Feeling supported, loved and encouraged can make all the difference in the decisions we make for our future, especially those related to changing our lifestyle. Sometimes it's necessary for us to review the support we have from others, and also realize we can reshape relationships and our personal world to help us flourish. This also allows you to be true to your personality and how you want to grow. Who are the five people closest to you? Do you look up to them? Do they inspire you? What do you enjoy about them? Do they make you feel supported and loved, and how do you even define these words? We often choose to see in people as subconscious recognition of ourselves. If you are choosing to see something in others, does it reflect something back to you about who you are or the kind of person you are being? You can do whatever you want and be whoever you want to be. What or who might you be allowing to stop you? Write down the qualities you would like to find in others when it comes to a support system and focus on how you can embrace these to attract the same attributes.

Gotta Love

These same questions can be asked regarding the relationship with yourself. How much do you love yourself? In our society we rush through our days and are so focused on the checklists, we forget to do anything that could nourish ourselves. With all the temporaries this world has to offer—moments, material things, relationships with others—the relationship with ourselves is permanent and we live with who we are every day. We will also remain unable to compassionately fill up someone else's cup if our cup remains empty. Of course, there will be times we feel drained, but what if taking an opportunity to check-in with ourselves daily allowed us to be happier the majority of time? It would at least give us a chance to make the choice as to what emotions we want to partake in and how we can set the tone for the time in front of us.

What emotions are you carrying? Where did they come from? How are they preventing you from moving forward? This can be parents, friends, that teacher that humiliated you in 6th grade. It's not to say that everyone is wrong in their actions, but sometimes individuals with the best intent come off in a fashion that gets misinterpreted by us in youth. It's coming to realize this that can be the most difficult. Communication can be strenuous and we all communicate differently. I'm sure you have experienced someone at some point in your life that you could by no means 'pick up what they were throwing down', regardless as to how hard you tried. Sometimes it's also because they did intend for it to be interpreted negatively or hurt you, but this goes back to their projection of pain.

This is where I would take the opportunity to sit in the sunshine on the patio and allow myself to journal. Most of us can benefit from writing things out or voice recordings if that's what you have time for, because this action in itself of describing how we are feeling and what's affecting us is moving that emotional energy out of our body and into the world. Write down the events, the people associated with them, how you feel about them today and your understandings as to why they did what they did. Commit to this no longer inhibiting your life.

How to Save a Life
The most important person to forgive in all of this…yourself. Releasing these pent up feelings will save your life. Many of us will go through this process and then sit there beating ourselves up wondering why we held onto these emotions for so long, watching days go by while we threw ourselves the pity party of a lifetime. This is just another distraction and a way of preventing the vision for our future. Know that you did the best you could at that time with what you knew. Most importantly, figure out what did you learn from these situations? There are negative habits that can develop from hurt, but there is also a lot of good. This is another way to focus your control in a perception, versus the lack of control you have in situations. How did these experiences make you stronger? What did they teach you about yourself and adaptations that need to take place? Which great personality traits that you carry with you today were shaped due to past events? Everything really does happen for a reason, and accepting that you are continuously growing and learning, will help to tap into those hidden talents and motivators, rather than ruminating on the bullshit.

Growing Pains
What did you love as a kid? A big part of our growing pains can be disconnecting from that child-like innocence. Brainstorm what this looked like and decide on some of those small things you can incorporate in to your life. If you have a family and are thinking "yeah right, when do I have time?", how could you integrate the two? Maybe your kids would love to feel closer to you by participating in something together, and it also allowing

them a deeper understanding of who you are. In whatever way, taking the time to reconnect with yourself will start to create an emotionally healthy thought process. Reinvigorating this love for the youthful version of yourself, reconnects you to that heart energy of happiness and joy, which is healing in itself. Then, rather than hyper-focusing on a 'to-do' list and what exists around us we can live in the moment. Which leads me to my next point...it's time to fill up your solo cup.

SUMMARY

Taking a hard look at our perspective and analyzing it in a way to improve our future, can sometimes be a disheartening reality check. At the same time that's a perspective in itself. Think of it as a way to better understand who you are and how your experiences have molded you into an art form. Just as the sun shines after the night falls, there is light that comes from journeying through the dark. When we discover ourselves and how we can encourage changes through improving our relationships, forgiveness, acceptance, and releasing expectations, the heavier times in our lives allow for a much greater appreciation as to what is. Take the good from all of the situations presented to you and utilize those learnings that you hold closest to your heart to ignite the fire within. Sometimes what we consider to be our biggest hurts, fears, and regrets, were meant to be this lifetime's biggest successes based on what we do with the information we have.

Chapter 3: Fill Up Your Solo Cup

*H*ow emotionally fulfilled is your 'cup'? As in YOU. That beautiful freaking being that needs to retrace its drops, so it can recognize the same. The only cup we need to worry about, is ours. If our solo cup is rim full, we will have much more to give and we are the only ones that can pour into it since we are responsible for US.

Now that we've discussed improving the relationships around you, and forgiveness to free yourself, what actions can we continue taking to love ourselves consistently so this concept blooms? Treating yourself is so often associated with outside things and materialism, and sometimes we need that, too! But emotionally staying in tune with ourselves doesn't have to involve a lot of dolla dolla bills.

Outside of scheduling time to play, staying positive and in the right frame of mind can be difficult. On a daily basis we are exposed to the complainers at work, the news that exaggerates the bad and leaves out most of the good, and the bickering on social media. We want to believe we can avoid feeding into these black holes, but exposure is everything. If you are not doing something to stay in a positive mindset surrounded by a world of blame and hate that constantly looks for ways to separate us as human beings, you will unknowingly fall victim. Even if you are someone who considers themselves very aware, it's too difficult to focus on awareness all the time when we have so many things going on around us.

MY DETOX

I personally do not watch the news much anymore. It had an intensely negative effect on me, and so did social media. I never understood how detrimental this was until I actively cut it out for a couple of weeks. All of a sudden, fear didn't strike simply by walking out the front door as it did when they were a part of my everyday life. Then I changed my social media feeds to follow people and articles that inspire me. If I feel I want to check in on what's going on in the world, I will read *The Skimm*, which is a digital publication that gets sent directly to my email. This isn't meant to come across as if I don't care about the world around me, it's actually quite the opposite. We are often given only a small amount of the truth, and the influence that creates fear-based thinking is not empowering for self-improvement, or understanding worldly events.

Next, I integrated a gratitude practice. Before, I had focused on the negative, due to hearing so much of it. But I figured out the trick. I set a phone calendar reminder for the morning and evening that simply says "Gratitudes and Goals." Before I get out of bed in the morning, I am already on a positive track. Even if I don't have time to physically write them, I list five things in my head that I am grateful for in the moment. After integrating this habit, I felt more content and recognized the gifts of the everyday, embracing my decisions and actions in a more thoughtful way. It actually changes the neural pathways in the brain! On top of it, when that jerk cuts me off in traffic later in the day, I say "May the force be with you," versus forcing a particular finger in the air. So, everyone wins with gratitude practice! The little things no longer get to me as much, and it's important to note that this internal stress shifts our immune system. Therefore, it's not just our mood we are improving, it's our entire physical being.[7]

Meditation was a train I was not willing to hop on initially, more less because I felt everything else was more important to get done. But after starting with some guided mediations via YouTube and an app, I became hooked! I felt so relaxed and many of the meditations I did were visualizations, so on top of being more present for ten minutes, I also had a sense of excitement when thinking about the future. Those visualizations even began to manifest, so it became more than self-care, but a way to go within and energetically take part in what my soul needed. Some days I will still have difficulty making time, but even on those days I will incorporate some deep breathing, which can be done anywhere. If you see me in public with a puffed-out stomach and red cheeks, I'm most likely deep breathing on the fly.

Whether it be just for a few minutes, when you scribe your emotions and why you are feeling the way you do, and or notate any physical pains or sensations, journaling and being present even in the slightest can allow us to become more in tune with ourselves and bodies. This helps us address things head-on rather than allowing them to fester. One of the things I have noticed in my own physical detoxification is how attuned I have become to my own body by incorporating regular check-ins. I can tell you the minute a muscle is out of alignment, or what foods will benefit me today, or what supplement I need. I never would have imagined my body could communicate to me on this level, but the intuition we can have is related to us slowing down and allowing it to speak. How many of us have an ache or pain and power through our day anyway, then forget about it later? Maybe the body is trying to tell you something and you are ignoring it. All the more reason to keep a scrolling note on your phone, or have access to a notebook so you can at least come back to it later.

Goal setting is another favorite way to begin the day. There are always too many things to do and too little time, right? Wrong. Think abundantly and tell yourself that there is plenty of time and see how your day changes. It's how we prioritize our important time that sets us up for success. As I set a reminder in my gratitude practice to write down goals, I choose the top three things, or some days just one thing, that I absolutely want to accomplish. This always changes for me, but we have to acknowledge our wins, and avoid counting our losses. I know in my healing process there were some days I was so exhausted that trying to force myself to check responsibilities off a list wasn't in me. Although it frustrated me feeling I was always tired and wasn't getting anything done, I also knew that forcing myself to do things I did not have the energy for would also drain me. Days like that, just making my bed was an accomplishment.

Affirmations have been an incredible addition to my life as well. Affirmations are what we believe true of who we are and what we deserve. As I mentioned one of my personal beliefs about myself in feeling "not good enough," I had to create affirmations proving this theory incorrect, such as "I am always enough". Sometimes washing away years of conditioning and negative self-talk can seem like a mountainous ascent. The good thing is there are two sides to every mountain, and by continuing our hypothetical climb, we will find a path that eases us back down in returning to a stronger more healed version of ourselves.

YOUR DETOX

Are you ready to make time for self-care? When we are so used to the opposite, sometimes self-care can feel like quite an intimidating animal to take on. The upside to this is whether it's baby steps or giant leaps, there are always options on how you can incorporate it daily. Either is a perfect way to start, because we will all find ourselves at different places in life at different times. Starting to make a change in your day no matter how big or small is the first step to getting results. Here are some suggestions that can offer you a place in the sun. See how you feel after a week and go from there. Once we try different avenues, we can begin to tap in to what works best for us and sometimes this is different things on different days.

Overexposed

Controlling our environment when it comes to what we see and hear might be difficult to do 100 percent of the time, but we can observe the constants in each day, and determine what role we can take in this. What social outlets are you using most and do you feel yourself uplifted by them, or in a state of constant comparison and wanting more? Decide which pages or people are most inspiring for you to follow. Who would you want to be friends with or which companies, brands and people do you want to support in areas you are most passionate about? Keep resonating with the feeling. Take some time to cut little things like this out to assist you in putting a positive spin on some of your consistent exposure to the outside world. This creates a healthier vibe that becomes the new norm.

Thankful

When do you feel most connected with yourself and your being? What helps you relax and feel at peace? It's easy for us to get distracted with what's going wrong around us because it's something we've been taught and what the general population leans to. We're even marketed to by companies in the mentality of there's always something better. Want a date? Swipe left or right and the moment a miscommunication comes up, run back to the app. But what if we quit searching for more, and we were content with everything we have?

Every day we wake up is a success. Our extraordinarily resilient bodies take in oxygen and pour it through us, so we can touch, taste, smell, see, and hear. Have you ever stopped and taken in all the senses you encounter in a moment? There is no guarantee for tomorrow, so appreciate what you have and the growth you've persevered through. A couple of minutes in recognizing what you are grateful for can go a long way. Start your morning with a list of five and witness how giving thanks for what is, creates more abundance. When we are content and grateful for something as little as the sun shining on our skin or as big as the promotion at work, we begin to quit searching therefore lessening the resistance that creates more of it. Being grateful for who you are is important as well, so be sure to throw in some affirmations that would be important in how you want to tap into your true essence. Affirmations can be any statements starting with 'I am' to improve how you embrace who you are and the mindset around it.

Oasis

Sometimes the things we resist the most are exactly what we need. Can you relate when it comes to meditating specifically? But if we take a few minutes to overlook the external chaos, there is an internal oasis. Meditation helps in remaining more present, enhances deep breathing (more oxygen benefits everything in our body) and it has been linked to increasing serotonin, which was that biochemical my body was inhibited in producing.[8] Serotonin keeps us cool, calm and collected, also converting to melatonin in the evening, which encourages our sleep cycle. If we are in "fight or flight" anxiety most of the day, which promotes stress hormones, our bodies can stay in that state and make it difficult to wind down at night, hence less restful sleep. Take time to slow down.

Deep breathing you can do anywhere once you get accustomed to it. There are a couple breathing patterns I utilize the most, one being the 4-7-8 breath. Breathe in through your nose for four seconds, hold the air in your lungs deep in the belly for 7 seconds, and then breathe pushing the air out through your mouth for 8 seconds. The other is in fives- 5 seconds in, 5 second hold, and 5 second breath out. Repeating these at least a few times in a row will help relax and promote beneficial chemical balances for your body and brain. It also helps to strengthen our primary respiratory muscles like the diaphragm under the ribs, which become weakened over time from the shallow breathing created by stress. It's my belief that we also decided looking skinny was more important than the "fat" look deep breathing offers. C'mon people! Breath is life. Let's make oxygen filled bellies a hashtag and change the world.

Dear Diary
Journaling is a quick way to release emotions and check in with yourself. A few minutes of writing here and there can give you a chance to stop, reflect, and be present as to what you are feeling. Whether it be physical or emotional, it all goes hand-in-hand. What events immediately come to mind when you think about the day or previous days? What feelings bubble up alongside these? Jot these along with what sensations you notice in your body as you are processing it all. Sometimes we can actually feel a release of tension in particular areas as we move our emotions internally through pen to paper. In this case, you can begin to see what kinds of emotions tend to get clustered in specific areas of your body. Just as I mentioned anger and resentment in the liver, this can also vary from person to person. Take note emotionally and physically how your body and mind are getting long together.

Along with hitting the breaks with this form of self-care, you could also write down goals and accomplishments. Goals can be anything for the day, week, month or next ten years. Vision boards are always a fun addition to thoughts around goals to spark some creative flow. Understanding why you are creating goals is also essential. As for accomplishments, I reflect on upon these at night-time when my gratitude reminder pops up again as a nice way to end my evening. It can be tempting to lay in bed and think about what we wish had gotten done during the day rather than everything we did complete. There are going to be days events detour our planned paths and we won't complete everything we goal ourselves to do. Rather than expecting, have the intention that it will get done while also realizing that not everything plays out the way we want it to. With everything happening for a reason, have you ever been glad that something didn't turn out the way your mind's eye envisioned? Maybe there's a series of events that will lead to a better outcome rather than what we originally intended for ourselves. Maybe you needed a lesson to come about in order to complete a goal at your highest potential.

SUMMARY

Today's "to dos" become more task and work oriented, but if you were happier because you included time for yourself in the day, would your life be easier? Your conversations more seamless? Make some time to treat yourself. This can be supportive on an emotional level, and in turn you'll feel it on the physical level. When you reflect on your accomplishments in the evening, put your self-care at the top of the list. Treating ourselves is also treating others, because they benefit from the flow of our happiness. This is not a box that we are creating with walls that will need to be broken down later such as previously mentioned conditioning. It's more of a blank canvas and you get to pick the colors that express the life you want.

Which of these self-care methods resonates with you? Try a sampler plate and see which ones make you feel the best. Whether it's a quick five minutes every morning and evening, a once a week hour of journaling, or maybe you have forty-five minutes a day and do a little of each. Trying to implement too many things at once can get overwhelming, so if you feel like you're more consistent in specific areas, utilize those as your daily regimens and integrate others once a week or month. Some of us have a little catching up to do in the self-love department, so as I heard in yoga class once, "keep your eyes on your own mat" and let's respect the time each of us needs as we have taken on different experiences to get us here. Some of us may need an hour a day to really create a pivotal force, where others can feel satisfied in a matter of minutes.

CHAPTER 4: WHAT THE FOOD?

*F*ifty years ago, we didn't understand the level of change our food went through chemically and otherwise by food producers and manufacturers. The USDA was influenced by lobbyists, and still is today. Did you know that's actually how the food pyramid came to be? It's not the servings everyone requires, but a paid advertisement by your commercial meat, dairy, grain, and other industries.[9] In addition to this, the FDA is also funded primarily by pharmaceutical companies. With one of their many responsibilities being ensuring the safety of our food supply as well as many other ingestible products, you can now imagine the more drugs that are sold, the more disposable money the FDA has available.[10] Don't get me wrong, there is a time and place for medication, and science and research are a beautiful thing, but that seems to be our first answer to everything, and I never want to hear of over-prescribing for the purpose of money. According to www.topmastersinhealthcare.com, in 2011 the average number of prescriptions per American was 13, and in 2013, www.statista.com reported this rising to 19.2. That's proof that we are overprescribing, and that people's bodies are having issues elsewhere when bandaged in one area versus corrected.

Greek Physician Hippocrates wrote way back in the day, "Food is medicine." The downside of today's foods is being brought to our attention. We are at a point in our society that people have accumulated so much damage from years of processed, chemically laden foods, and meats that contain antibiotics and hormones, they either stay committed to what seems to be weekly doctors' appointments and multiple prescriptions, or they decide to start making changes by eating organic and hope to correct the root of the cause. I am not saying one is wrong, I only hope that people can see the alternative route of healthier foods, but we must make these decisions for ourselves and our state of mind.

Our society tends to make things more complicated as we continue to look outside ourselves for answers rather than in. It's important to begin to trust ourselves with what fits our health best. In this case, what we literally put in our bodies can be the answer to a lot of problems. Fruits and vegetables have qualities that can help bind to toxins that have accumulated and move them out. They also offer protective antioxidants and phytonutrients—dependent on the color of the food—and these protect us on a cellular level from free radical damage. Free radicals in our body are unstable atoms or molecules that have a free electron, making them highly reactive and capable of taking things from us we may need to absorb. These guys can develop from stress, eating processed meats, taking medications, pollutants in the air...You name something that's not biologically compatible with what already exists in our body, and it can most likely offer up a free radical of some kind. Even healthy foods can break down incorrectly, depending on the cooking methods, and create free radicals. Steaming veggies, for example, is a great way to make them easier to digest, while adding the hydration of water and maintaining their nutritional integrity. In saying this, our body does have an amazing ability to heal itself, but why test its capacity? We never know how much is too much until something significant arises, so should we wait until disease is upon us to find out, when we already know we can control what goes down the hatch?

MY DETOX

Anytime I saw the always repulsive pea circling my steak as a kid, I cringed. I ate a pretty standard diet growing up, with my favorite cinnamon toast crunch cereal for breakfast, the turkey sandwich with miracle whip mayonnaise (damn, I loved that stuff! I even ate it out of the jar.), the anticipated fruit roll-up buried in the 'My Little Pony' acrylic lunch box, or even better- a Hostess cupcake. Dinners always involved a meat, veggie, and starch. Let's pray we have some chocolate ice cream while I watch "Walker Texas Ranger" tonight! This was being healthy then.

As I got older, entering middle school and the land of the bullies, I became more active in sports and more interested in health food choices. The problem with my definition of it was that it stemmed from a body image problem. I started only eating when I was hungry, and would push this as far as I could. I wanted that desirable slender physique, just like the girls on Teen Magazine. I was too judgmental of myself to realize I already had it. In high school, I ate a lot more fruits and veggies, spacing out snacks similarly to how I eat today. Working out and playing field hockey needed a different kind of fuel if I didn't want to get sick mid-sprint. This continued to evolve as I went into college. I began food-prepping in my mid-20s, but there were still the budget-friendly ramen noodles that came into play from time to time. Although I was eating incredibly healthy compared to the Hostess cake trades at the middle school lunch table, there were still changes that needed to be made knowing now how they caught up with my physical toxicity.

So, what is healthy? Everyone thinks they have the next best diet in which the entire population would benefit from. As I dealt with diet through my personal health Olympics, I felt this was a subject in which I already excelled. In the few years leading up to it, I cut out all of gluten and dairy, watched my corn intake as I noticed that it was hard on my digestive tract, and the only sugars I would partake in were local raw honey and maple syrup, if a healthy muffin recipe called for it. This needed to be cut out for a while too, because although there's a great mineral profile in these condiments, there's still a high sugar content.

Turns out there's a whole lot more to what we put in our bodies than the guidelines we believe are healthy. Even though some of what I was eating at the time might be excellent for me in my near future, the toxins my body was trying to process in that moment would feed a bacteria overgrowth in the gut, as well as parasites. It became incredibly frustrating as I continued to cleanse my liver, the toxins fed bacteria, so parasite cleansing had to occur and then repeat. I had a test done to analyze the type of bacteria that were overgrown, and then I started a low FODMAP diet. FODMAP is an acronym referring to short chain carbohydrates that are difficult to digest in the small intestine (Fermentable Oligo-saccharides, Di-saccharides, Mono-sac-charides And Polyols). Some bacterial strains will feed off of the early fermentation of these foods (since they are not getting broken down as soon as they should), encouraging a dysbiosis, or more of one if it already exists. A dysbiosis, is when the good bacteria and bad bacteria in the gut are out of balance, typically with the bad team winning. We all have a little bit of both but maintaining the balance between the two is key to healthy digestion, and an entirely healthy body for that matter.

This diet didn't seem to make me feel my best, so then I tried GAPS, which stands for Gut and Psychology Syndrome. This diet encourages the elimination of specific foods that supposedly effect the bacteria in the gut negatively, causing neurological symptoms like ADHD, anxiety, depression, etc. These foods exclude most carbohydrates, while encouraging the consumption of meats, veggies, and fermented foods. In many cases the diet also removes fruits for a while due to the sugar content.

What I learned through my process, was that no pre-pre-scribed diet worked for me. I ended up researching the bacteria strains and what they thrived on. This gave me some insight and confirmed why these diets were not working. Just because a food would become associated with breaking down early on in the digestive tract, did not mean that was the case for my body. Fermented foods can sometimes feed negative bacterial strains too, depending on your unique bacterial profile, so it worsened my situation. There are still many bacterial strains to be discovered, so although this is an important area of research, it's safe to assume that what has been discovered is not the end all be all, and also not applicable to every person. The only cravings I did have to be leery of were carbohydrates and grains. Candida (which is a yeast in our body), bacterial strains, and parasites thrive on too many of these and sometimes craving these means they want it, not you. Candida is supposed to be there, but when it too becomes overgrown, digestive complications can occur.

On top of all this, I also did some genetic testing and the toxicity caused an issue with a gene that helps to remove excess sulfurs from the body. If you cannot remove all the sulfurs from foods, it can then turn into ammonia that damages the nervous system. Here I was thinking I was eating so well by including broccoli and cauliflower in my diet, but it turns out there was a reason that I was sort of repulsed by the looks of them when I was in the produce aisle—they're higher in sulfurs. I normally love these foods, but I had no desire for them. I forced it because I thought they were good for me and my body needed all the nutrition it could get. The minute I cut out all cruciferous vegetables, garlic and onion, my skin cleared some and so did a lot of my fatigue, brain fog, and chronic pain. All foods are going to have sulfur in them to some extent, but the ones highest in it can create an overload for those with what's called a CBS gene mutation (knowing whether it's up-regulated or down-regulated is important for those of you that have it).

I fell victim to the idea that restrictions were healthy even at a young age. Like many of us do, I became incredibly self-conscious of my outward appearance. Looking back, it hurts me to think my eighth-grade self was worried her thighs were too big. I began to weigh myself regularly, worked out like crazy, and some days I would feel so down on myself that I would eat as little as my parents would let me get away with. Health became very skewed in my world, and rather than wondering if my body had the fuel it needed, or focusing on what my body could do, I was concerned with clothing size, weight, and the number of calories I took in.

Fast forward into adulthood- I carried this over into being obsessive about numbers in relation to calories and macros. I would use apps to count every numerical value related to the food that went into my mouth. If I cooked something at home, I would add up the calories, fats, carbs, and proteins of all the ingredients, and then calculate those values per serving size. The amount of time I spent focused on my food was becoming overwhelming, while I was missing the biggest factor of all. Was what I was eating even good for my body? And do calories even matter if I'm eating to satiety and incorporating whole foods? Emotionally, I was dealing with a lot of fear and control issues that were unmeasurable outside of a Fitbit and I had no idea what to do with them.

Counting calories also doesn't mean you're not full of... sugar. When I worked in an office in the past, I was a frequent visitor to the colorful candy bowl which I believe was strategically placed within 3 feet of my desk. I stole all the pink Starbursts (I just gave myself up to any previous coworkers potentially reading this), loved the mini Reece's cups, and was happy to head to the vending area for a Dr. Pepper, I typically referred to as a 'DP'. This is not only an immensely large amount of sugar, it's incredibly hard on the liver and bloodstream. Our pancreas works hard to balance our blood sugar, and excess glucose is stored in the liver as glycogen for back-up energy. So, I not only had the glucose circulating in my bloodstream, I had major back-ups in the form of a SWAT team, Navy Seals, and the CIA taking post in my liver, ready to act if I needed them. Most of us do this, then wondering why we want to pass out at our desks around 3pm.

Although diets, numbers, and attentiveness to my physical appearance did not work for me long-term, it all led me to my own conclusion: intuitive eating is when we literally trust our guts in guiding us to the food our body needs to function properly. I realized rather than trying to look outside of myself for answers, all the answers I needed were staring back at me in the mirror every morning. I was refusing to listen, because it becomes difficult to break the habit of maintaining a perspective that is influenced by society and "experts." How unsuccessful would health and wellness advocates be if all we had to do was intuitively eat and avoid strict diet guidelines? I feel we should never assume we know it all nor play by someone else's rules until we have done some self-analysis. No matter what the subject matter. It's also important to understand what other factors in our life- such as my mentioned control issues- might be interfering with us letting go and flowing with what our body needs. Now by trusting my gut, I am physically healthier, my fitness fell into place, and I'm in the best shape of my life, all while not worrying how my body looks to others and causing my own anxiety.

YOUR DETOX

Foods

I can sit here and discuss the different nutritious qualities of each fruit and vegetable all day long. Besides the fact that it would be boring as hell for the majority of people reading this, all the little details won't add up to what the dietary changes will do for you in the long run. With quality as the focus, you can change so much more in regard to your health and longevity.

First off, in choosing foods, look for antibiotic and hormone free. Hormones are given to female cows to regulate lactation and reproduction, and antibiotics are given to animals to prevent or remedy illness so they can still be utilized as a food source. Antibiotics, however, are manmade and some these chemicals can get stored in the tissues which we eat. Hormones can also get passed from the animal to us by drinking their milk, and have been linked to cancers like breast, prostate and endometrial.[11] Our bodies don't require the antibiotics and hormones getting passed down from our foods, and they can upset our natural chemistry.

This also includes antibiotic resistance, which is contributing to a lot of health issues as antibiotics kill good bacteria too, effecting our immune system and our genes negatively. These bacterial changes are then passed on to our youth through the placenta and uterine wall, which is why we are seeing an increase in many cases of food allergies, juvenile diabetes and neurological complications. The majority of bacteria is held in our gut which is often referred to as the microbiome, consisting of about 70-85% of our immunity.[12] Unhealthy bacterial strains then also learn how to survive by adapting to our internal environment and mutating to bypass antibiotics, becoming harder for us to kill. If the good bacteria is too low to do anything about this in order to balance the scales, which is again referred to as a dysbiosis, it can lead to sickness becoming more difficult for us to recover from or stave off. Eating foods containing antibiotics and hormones here and there won't hurt us immediately, but all of this adds up as time goes on, so it's best to cut it out before you're faced with a health crisis that becomes difficult to reverse.

Moving on to the next best quality of meat, in addition to

antibiotic and hormone-free, look for non-GMO, indicating the food given to the animal was not genetically modified. The main reason plants were changed on a genetic level to begin with was to withstand different seasons so they could be available year-round. If we were modified so that we could wear jean shorts and tank tops all year, even in the winter, I would be concerned, regardless of my love for both of these fashion staples. So, animals we consume are eating a somewhat imposter of a seed. For instance, the corn given to chickens may not have been organic, but it was non-GMO, so therefore the chicken cannot be organic because of the food it consumed. The corn was not biologically manipulated in creating the seed, but it was sprayed with pesticides and herbicides. Hence, if you find organic meats, they have been given organic or unsprayed feed, and the source of that feed was not manipulated on a genetic level.

When it comes to beef, people that look for the highest quality will purchase organic, grass-fed, and pasture raised. This guarantees that the meat is organic, the cows ate their natural food source, and they were humanely raised. There are theories that if an animal suffered, the painful energy that the animal experienced can be transferred to the person eating it. It may sound a little wild to most of us, but if you are around your best friend and they are in a funk one day, do you feel it? We all have a level of emotional intuition even if we have not quite committed to recognizing it on an intimate level. Take from this what you will.

"Eat the rainbow" is becoming a common phrase amongst the healthy food community. It's referring to all the antioxidants and phytonutrients reflected in the form of color. The thought is if we make sure to incorporate all the colors we take in at the grocery store or farmer's market, we will be fully supported in what our body needs nutritionally. Choosing organic when you can, is the best bet for fruits and veggies as well, but there is a list called "the dirty dozen" which can be utilized as a guide. This list is referring to inorganic fruits and vegetables that are the "dirtiest," or have the highest amount of detectable pesticides, and "clean," which have the lowest amount. If you are looking to watch your chemical intake, but also manage a budget, this list will help guide you in buying organic for the most contaminated fruits and vegetables, while knowing you can get conventionally grown for the cleaner produce.

It can be difficult when families grow to maintain a fully organic kitchen because of the expense, if you were lucky to even have one in the first place. There are also indications out there of organic being less nutritious than non-organic foods because of the soil changes. What's the point in eating a vegetable if you aren't going to receive any health benefits? This is one reason buying organic can be expensive. With all the chemically effected farmland, it can take quite a bit of work for a farm to turn that over and begin again as organic, enriching the soil as it should be. This becomes a hardship for farmers alongside the rising demand, factoring in other agricultural components I can hardly imagine. They have laborious enough jobs and encounter difficulties in maintaining business due to large scale commercial competitors.

Many pesticides work so that when consumed, they poke holes in the stomachs of bugs and they die. We may not be 100% compatible with the genetics of a bug, but we are all carbon-based beings, and I find it interesting in paralleling this with the amount of people affected with leaky gut. This is when there are gaps in the intestinal walls that food leak through and get into the blood stream. This can cause a whole host of health problems, as you then have floating particles in places they shouldn't be.

You might be wondering: do the previous paragraphs mean I have to give up chocolate? Absolutely not! I eat dark chocolate many a days, and if there were lobbyists advocating for that as part of our food pyramid, I could be convinced to pay more taxes. It's full of antioxidants which will combat those free radicals, and it's delicious! 70% cacao or higher is the best, alongside having less sugar. Just like there are quality meats, fruits, and veggies, look for the same in your snacks. There are a lot of great options out there, as the popularity and creativity are flowing with gluten free, vegan, and organic options. It's definitely better to include mostly fruits and vegetables in your diet of course, but you can find some nutrition in premade options these days without feeling restricted or less connected to your inner foodie.

Having that glass of wine on occasion or nachos at the ballgame will not hurt you enough to reverse a normally consistent healthy lifestyle. It's learning to manage it so you're not over indulging on a regular basis. Going with the theme of energy as well, if you are excited to eat something and it's connecting you to your joy, give yourself the space to indulge as your body will process it better than if you are guilting yourself. Make the best choices you can the majority of time, yet also find the trust in yourself to balance your happiness with health.

Numbers
But wait-how many calories is that? Calories, counting steps,

carbs, fats and proteins-oh my! There are so many things to keep track of. Fad diets are on the rise as well as the many devices to measure our "macros." There are definitely benefits here to counting and macros as they both make us more aware of what we are putting in our body, the calories in versus calories out and the number of steps we average. However, I've met many people with a similar anxiety to mine that has been created by the manic focus these can create. The teaching mechanism can be excellent, but when we notice ourselves taking this too far, then we need to set them aside for a while. Anything can be addictive regardless of intent, so just as we need to put our cell phones away for a day here and there, we need to do the same when these healthy tools go from beneficial to detrimental.

Our bodies are giant chemistry projects and they will speak for us if we allow it. Biochemistry may not be your expertise, nor is it mine, but in realizing that the chemical make-up of my body is what is driving cravings, it has become a powerful fitness tracker on its own. It also allowed me to feel better and eliminate toxins more quickly. If we make sure bacteria and parasites are not part of the equation first, then we can decipher that the craving is something our body truly needs. When I had heavy cravings for sugar and starch, I knew that was due to the yeast and bacteria needing to be balanced. Since this had been addressed to some extent, I knew when I began craving peanut butter next, it was because the arginine in it worked to process some excess ammonia in my body. I had a couple of weeks where I couldn't keep my spoon out the jar. I was walking around like Brad Pitt in *Meet Joe Black*. All of a sudden, the craving disappeared. In saying all of this, remain focused on what your body is craving. You may want to research the foods you crave, but if you are eating a healthy, quality diet with clean meats and mostly organic veggies, your body will get everything it needs when you hear it out. Hopefully you don't have to purchase as much stock in the peanut butter industry as I did.

Many times, we feel as if cutting these tasks out will make us gain weight and create a lack of control. There is a level of aligning with your goals, but no matter what those are, by letting go of the numbers we will actually gain more control. In fact, we typically lose weight, feel better, and with this comes freedom. If your goal is being healthier, you become more aware of how you feel with certain foods, learning what fits your body and chemistry best. If your goal is letting go of controlling body image issues, you can begin to release the control on how to connect more with your joy in this process versus being potentially drained by a regimen. The perception again is restrictive in and of itself when we 'think' we must eliminate foods, calories or macros. There is no such thing unless we create it. Allow by allowing, and although it make take some getting used to and potential emotional healing alongside it, the end result is much more fulfilling, self-accepting, and less time consuming.

Sugar
So, what is the big deal with sugar then? Is this something we should flow with? Sugar has been linked to inflammation in the body, which can encourage genes that have been linked to diseases and of course they effect the amount of insulin released in our blood stream along with the accumulation of fat. You may notice an increase in the number of people with Type 2 diabetes, which

is often times related to the consumption of sugar, however this can be controlled or even reversed. Type 1 diabetes is when the pancreas is under-producing insulin, creating inflammation and stress on the pancreas, while glucose then fluctuates in the bloodstream. Thus, Type 1 diabetics need to be on insulin to maintain its function, and prevent other organs from distress that it holds a relationship with. Insulin is what is released when we need absorption of the glucose or sugar into cells for energy. With Type 2 diabetes, if the pancreas becomes overworked due to excess sugar intake, there's not enough insulin to take care of the amount of glucose in the blood stream, which can lead to an excess amount being stored in the liver. The pancreas also has other functions including hormonal support and the secretion of digestive enzymes, so if one area is exhausted, it can affect its function elsewhere. If you eat a donut for breakfast with tons of sugar, your body works overtime to control the amount of sugar that's being released into the blood. The pancreas ups its game but becomes very focused and distracted on this one of many responsibilities.

Glucose is what many sugars are broken down into, and it's also what is burned as fuel. Now, your body needs energy to do simple tasks such as blink and breathe, but if you go to work and sit all day, there's not enough blinking you could do to burn all the glucose you took in from that delectable donut. The excess glucose in our blood then gets stored in the liver as glycogen, and when we do use up what glucose is available for energy in the blood stream, our body will say "open sesame," and the liver offers the back-up. For the Standard American Diet, which unfortunately is also abbreviated as "SAD," we typically don't stop at one donut. We have sugary snacks throughout the day, and dessert after dinner. This influx of sugar, break in eating, then influx of more sugar, is what makes us tired. It also breeds more sugar cravings because we've encouraged our body to need it as a normal rhythm, and as I mentioned, bacteria can sometimes be the ones behind our cravings.

Sugar also starts to become addictive as it activates the rewards center of our brain, and then we need it to get through the day. Our most important organ in detoxification, the liver, is trying to handle this load in addition to removing anything we don't want in our body, assimilating hormones, and hundreds of other things. If you had a task to do at work, would you feel stressed if your phone started ringing off the hook while your boss dropped off a stack of papers to review and a coworker across the office was instant messaging you with questions? Now you understand how our poor liver feels.

Breaking sugar cravings can be tough, but just like everything else, we need to start small. A lot of people will try to cut it all out immediately and often times fail. When we go too extreme too quickly, we stress ourselves out and it also sets us up to feel regretful of our action if we give in earlier than hoped. So instead of grabbing three Starbursts at a time at work, grab one. Rather than using white sugar in your coffee, try some honey. The trick is in the amount too, so eventually, use less and less if you are using them as a sweetener. Green leaf stevia is my favorite due to the fact it does not affect glucose levels and the whole leaf has numerous health benefits. If you feel like you are starving while shopping at the grocery store, grab an apple instead of a Snickers bar. The changes will gradually happen for you as your taste buds adapt, and this will allow you to be more successful while being compassionate to your body as it is able to slowly morph as well. Again, biochemistry is a part in all of this so it's not just our habits that are changing, it's our body on a cellular level.

When we go back to the subject of connecting with our joy and inner foodie, sugar is also a component of this. It's okay to allow ourselves the cheats, it's again finding a balance that works for you. If you are craving sugar all the time, then we have to detox the palette so you can understand when you are actually emotionally enjoying your food, versus biologically needing it to stay awake or functioning. There's a big difference!

SUMMARY

Detoxing your body to create cravings around healthier choices can take some time. With comparison and societal influences also playing a big part in food, I believe the hardest part for most of us is letting go of the control and taking the time to listen to our bodies' needs. It's all too common to base our habits off of what we see around us as opposed to what we feel is right.

This patience can be trying in a world of instant gratification, even with ourselves, but this is not social media. This is your body we are talking about. Your temple. Your vessel of life. Love it, listen to it and take your time with it. It will love you right back and stick with you if you do, and chances are you are setting yourself up for a more beautiful future than the past ever was or could have been. Our bodies get used to operating with foreign invaders and bad eating habits, just like it does prescription medications. Don't yank the rug out from under it too hard or too quickly. Be patient with your changes.

CHAPTER 5: GET A MOVE ON

Working out is also where we focus on digital helpers like fitness trackers, heart rate monitors and pedometers. Our bodies will let us know how much movement we have in us day to day, as it does with what it wants to eat. Through my experience this year and being forced to rethink my workouts, I realized that although they didn't feel as intense, walking was all I was physically capable of, outside of some stretching for about a month. I feel we forget to give ourselves enough credit or compassion when it comes to the amount of energy exerted in a day. At least when it comes to my routine, by the time I've taken care of my daily responsibilities, I'm already wiped out! Some days it feels like there's not a free moment to really sit down and enjoy the quiet. Other days I wake up and feel like I can take on the world with an hour-long workout. Now more than ever when I rise in the morning, I see how I feel, and adjust accordingly.

Many of us associate the amount we move with what we eat. Too often we overindulge in food and then feel that running five miles is going to offset that amount. But that's not how the body works. We think there's a quick fix for everything, including the relationship of food consumption to exercise. However, for as much energy there is in the food we devour, the same amount of energy is needed to remove it. Focusing on the aesthetics of working out takes us away from truly being healthy. We also look to workouts for guidance in a similar fashion as diets. We all have unique bodily compositions, hormonal balances, muscle fibers, and so on. Trusting your gut according to what energizes you and connects you to your happiness, is just as important in how we get a move on.

MY DETOX

I participated in nearly every sport and physical activity I can think of growing up. My mom often told people I was born with a ball in my hand. Exercise for me came naturally as I enjoyed the camaraderie and feeling physically empowered. I loved late summer nights, playing basketball in the backyard, jump roping with my friend across the street, or playing hopscotch in between catching fireflies. Cartwheels in the front yard were a regular thing as I did gymnastics in my youth. Eventually I dabbled in karate, track, volleyball, then field hockey in high school.

I started early in the weight room around 12 years old, as my dad showed me around, and I began to go with him period-ically following what he did. As my enjoyment in the gym grew, I started learning more and created my own workouts. As I mentioned earlier though, I also began to have body issues around this timeframe too from all the media and dealing with my female bullies. With all the exercise and athletic involvement I was already a part of as a kid, I began to become obsessive about it. I popped in workout videos at home in my spare time, in addition to all my extra-curriculars. Even though I have not had an experience in being overweight, I do have empathy to those with any kind of negative body issues because I under-stand how this can affect mental well-being and relationships.

As I moved into high school, I would join in on weight training sessions with the football team, along with a few other girls from field hockey. Although there was still some feeding of that overly perfectionistic physical attainment, I absolutely loved the environment and enjoyed quality time with my friends. I tended to establish friendships more easily with guys, seeing as I was so into sports. I didn't connect with girls as much, feeling less accepted by them in middle school and maintaining the thought process with age that they were "drama." I utilized this as a defense out of fear in getting hurt emotionally. The guys always supported me for who I was, and if we pissed each other off it was dealt with in a few minutes, continuing on with our lives. I adapted to some of their natures, including being competitive and incredibly active. Regardless as to some of the unhealthy reasons of comparison, it did have benefits in influencing my health today. Some of these moments also offered the best memories of my life.

I continued lifting weights as a young adult and played in recreational volleyball and football leagues. Having time to myself at the gym was therapeutic, while allowing me to feel strong and in control of my health. As the toxins took a toll on my body this past year, my muscles reflected the stress, as they began to feel stiff and immovable. It was as if every time I tried to do a workout, within a few repetitions my muscles would feel like they were in rigor mortis. This was so frustrating since movement was incredibly important in my life and plays a big part in who I am.

When I went to the doctor for the first time, I was told that because of these adrenal fatigue symptoms, I should stick with just going for walks until my energy returned. Adrenal fatigue can happen for several reasons, but it's essentially referring to the hormones like aldosterone, adrenaline, cortisol and others that influence our energy levels. If you feel exhausted all the time, it could mean you have stress in this area, and by adding more physical stress, even in the form of exercise, you can cause damage long-term. I didn't know whether to cry or throw a full-blown tantrum in anger. No medical offices' post-appointment lollipop would fix my dismay (nor could I have the sugar). Telling me to sit still was not something that set well with me, along with my despair in not understanding what was happening to my body. On top of it, I experienced what is referred to as "muscle wasting." Since my body's systems were affected on a number of levels, it took from my proteins and what strength I had built over time, slowly started to dwindle. This was too much!

I needed to reflect on why this was so upsetting. There was a part of me that enjoyed movement and its cathartic effects, however there was also a voice in me that required I go to the gym five times a week or more, and if I didn't abide, I would become overweight and undesirable. Wow! A wake-up call occurred. Unfortunately, although I would have preferred to learn this in an easier way, I never would have recognized those "or else" emotions. Why did I need the gym and a specific body type to feel desirable or approved of? And why did I need anyone to approve of me other than me? This detox continued to reveal unhealthy beliefs I took part in, which also needed an overhaul. Acting based on unhealthy beliefs is what steals our spirit, rather than simply doing things because we enjoy them.

Sometimes when we are forced to sit still, the most profound emotions bubble up and allow us to face our demons head on. I realized I was still carrying those negative body images from my youth and had to redefine what my workouts meant to me, not allowing them to resonate with any self-worth or outside approval of others. Many of us can become obsessed about the amount of time we spend at the gym, how much cardio we're doing, or calories we are burning to look acceptable to the general public. When we think about it, the purpose of working out has nothing to do with any of that. The purpose of working out is to move the blood, move the lymphatic system, increase oxygen intake, build lean muscle mass to support our bones, ligaments and tendons. It's for proper function and longevity. Just as everything else we are discussing in this detox process, I came to realize that inside the body was way more important than outside. In clearing everything out, it allowed me to connect to the biology of what is really happening during movement and how my emotions were getting in the way of truly enjoying it.

I had become unknowingly emotionally focused by comparing my body to the bodies of others and looking towards competitiveness to give me strength, versus tapping into my power in multiple other ways outside the gym. I had many other gifts that could have been nourished, but because of feeling inadequate and believing that looks were of higher importance, I avoided exercising those skills. We are all blessed with our uniqueness yet can become so concerned with all the opinions and aesthetic ideals of believing there is one perfect body type. Sometimes a downfall allows for the greatest growth, and in my case, it came in the form of exhaustion and hesitant long walks.

What do my workouts look like today? Yes, I definitely still go to the gym and lift weights about three or four times a week. Understanding my "why" is what is different. The length of time has changed too, as we only need 30 to 45 minutes per session, if that. I usually go to yoga once a week to increase flexibility and elongate my muscles, in opposition to weights shortening them. Sweating via a hot class allows my body to remove additional toxins that I may have accumulated in the meantime.

Yoga was also one of the few workouts that I was able to do while I was going through the heaviest piece of detoxification, so it holds a special place in my heart now versus why I did it a few years ago. When my body was warm from the heat in the room, it allowed my muscles to open more, softening the stiffness. It was also a form of cardio that wasn't quite as jarring as running. Nothing bad in the body can survive in an oxygen-rich environment, and our atmosphere is constantly degrading as pollution breaks it down. This can require us to look for other ways to increase it in our own lives, cardio workouts being one of them. Meditation and physical connectedness in yoga also helped me keep my sanity as I definitely had my ups and downs. Feeling depressed many days, I was doing my best to keep a positive mind frame focusing on the light at the end of this unfamiliar tunnel.

Another important lesson for me in reconnecting to my "why" in exercise, was recalling the joy I experienced as a kid. Out of all the sports I tried growing up, my favorite was gymnastics. I loved how that sport made me feel. Gymnastics combines strength and power, while integrating grace and femininity. This was beauty to me. I guess you could say it also helped me feel more confident in who I was, and the characteristics I chose to see in gymnastics were how I identified as being a female. I got tired of hearing societal opinions of women as the weaker sex, so in a way I used my physical strength to prove this theory wrong. Once again, there's no reason for us to have to prove our worth, but my identity in this sport helped develop who I am today and there's always something good that comes from every situation. Rejuvenating this piece of me via similarities in yoga and aerial arts, aided in my healing when I felt defeated otherwise.

I used to over work my body at times thinking I'd feel better about the junk food I planned on inhaling during the weekends. The flip side to this was it expedited my adrenal fatigue as I completely depleted my body through intensive group exercise, not to mention the fact that nutrition was where I should have focused, rather than calories. Having found a better balance, accepting my body void of aesthetic or caloric guilt, I hope your detox supports fitness goals to the same satisfaction.

YOUR DETOX

Free Bird

Why do you work out? Do you truly do it for yourself, or are you more worried about what other peoples' opinions might be? Do you work out too little or too much? One of the questions that helped me reconnect with why I work out is, "What did I enjoy when I was a kid?" Children play in a way that exerts a lot of energy—running, jumping, skipping—but is also so enjoyable that it lights them up. As we get older, we begin to smother that fire and look at exercising as a responsibility, and one more thing that needs to be checked off our list. What if you could find a way

71

to exercise regularly, reconnect with that lively spirit that used to love it, and feel more invigorated while looking forward to your workout? It could mean going to a nearby beach to surf, going to a mountain to bike, or a park for a run that will encourage you to reconnect with who you once were and still are. Or maybe taking a yoga class three times a week could bring up some emotional associations with youth. Take some time to think about what you really care about when it comes to exercise. How might you be able to incorporate past joys into your current experience to make you feel more free and happy? Decide the frequency and how this can fit into your schedule. Ask your friends to join you so you can get the workout in and catch-up or make a family-oriented event around a hike. Community and connectivity create a level of well-being that can add to the experience.

Balance

Rather than beating ourselves up about eating too many calories and how quickly the pounds needs to come off, we should look towards the future and how we can make changes that will slowly support our goals. If it's the occasional cheat meal, enjoy those calories as you take them in and recognize that it's okay to happily indulge. There's no need to do this and then punish yourself with workouts. That's what your brain will then begin to associate with working out...punishment. Saying we want to enjoy a cheat meal and then guilting ourselves the entire time we take it in is contradictory, as we are not actually fully enjoying it. Rather than focusing on the number, let's focus on the health of our body and mind together.

If you wake up one morning and your body says all I can do

is walk, then walk. Don't worry about calories in and calories out. If you've been in the car all day or sitting at your desk and are overwhelmed from the amount of stress at work, don't push yourself for 10,000 steps. Go to bed early and get the well-deserved rest your body needs, so it can have enough energy the next day to support you in whatever ways you need to be supported. Recognize the quality of foods you are consuming, and whether you're eating because of hunger or emotion. In becoming more aware, counting calories can become a thing of the past while you provide your body with what it needs, which will typically parallel to the amount you move. When we fight our bodies, they will fight us back. Too many headaches from this struggle can also preoccupy us with things that we would rather enjoy.

Have you ever had moments where everything seemed to be going wrong? Maybe this caused a lack of sleep multiple nights in a row? All of a sudden, we wake up sick because we avoided what our body tried to explain to us as we continued pushing through to live up to expectations in work and family duties. At a certain point, it's going to show you how to slow down, whether you listen to the tiredness and take a nap, or you push through stress and wake up sick. Move your body when you can, and listen to it when you can't. What actions are you drawn to and what is it telling you it needs? Don't wake up next weekend sick because your personal priorities are more important than what your body is prioritizing for you.

SUMMARY
The relationship and connection we have to our physical being,

will allow us to improve the relationship with ourselves as well. We become intuitively tapped in and get to a place of knowing what we need. We can scientifically dig and look to others as examples, but just like all the studies out there, we are complex beings and there are too many variables on an individual level. Sometimes we must let go of statistics and allow faith in ourselves and what we know, to drive us to the best health. Our body is our vehicle through life, and that is not a small task. It has our back. Literally.

CHAPTER 6: ANALYSIS PARALYSIS

*T*esting is great, but how much should we rely on it? Which ones are best for our situation? Number ranges and data can be supportive, but is it the end all be all? Analyzing our bodies in a detailed way to inquire if the engine is running smoothly can be a helpful tool. I went through a series of different tests, now holding a manila folder thick enough for a fine antique bookshelf. Looking outside ourselves even in the form of testing can disconnect us from what we are trusting in building the relationship with our body. Ask yourself, what's my intent behind testing and is it taking me away from trusting my own biology? There's no reason not to combine these two, so let's figure out how we can balance the scales.

MY DETOX
Feeling like the largest lab rat up for experimentation, I was exhausted from participating in so much testing. I often thought I should be placed in a maze, while people watched from above as I ran head-first into a bunch of walls to find my beloved cheese. All I wanted to do was get back to my badass cage and run on my wheel. Even though it was monotonous at times to feel like I had to deal with so much physical analysis, I was amazed at the amount and intensity of testing available through functional medicine and naturopathy.

The first test I did was your typical blood analysis. This gave us a place to start and helped identify any deficiencies I may have been dealing with. If there were multiple numbers out of whack, we could look at why this could be and how they might be interwoven. The lab you are getting results from may also determine your results. I realized immediately that in my blood test through naturopath care, I had different "normal" ranges compared to the tests I had done with my primary care physicians in the past. Sometimes the measurements that are tested and the quality in analyzing data comes down to money. Most decisions made surrounding testing comes down to insurance coverages and costs anymore. The problem with this is the cheaper options are typically not the most informative routes. Although naturopathy is not covered in my state, being able to understand these aspects of testing was worth the money. What if we were given more options rather than the lab choice being made for us? Sometimes there might be certain results that we personally feel are more of a priority in analysis, and we do have a right to make specific requests.

After receiving the results of my initial test, it was obvious my numbers were all over the place, especially my white blood cells. This lab did me the honor of color-coding the low, normal and high ranges in yellow, green and red. Let's just say I am glad there were only three-colors as identifiers, otherwise we may have had many a rainbows... White blood cells can be an indicator of bacteria and fighting off infection. Neutrophils are a white blood cell that can be indicative of bacteria overgrowth in the gut and elsewhere. Mine were very high, and this also depleted some of my other white blood cells, leaving me defenseless in different areas of the body.

Due to the fact I had the Paragard IUD, we investigated saliva testing to see what the hormone levels were and if it was connected to my digestion, muscle aches and pains, and fatigue. Although it helped to understand more on the subject, it was not the solution. The supplements I started were helping some, but they did not resolve my health. For those of you ladies out there having hormonal issues, saliva tests are available online and can be requested from the doc. This can help in the decision as to which birth control to choose if you do decide to take it. Some estrogens are linked to cancers if they are out of balance, so as much as we want to prevent pregnancy, there should be more clarity and understanding as to what could result in what we put our bodies through.[13]

Up next was testing for heavy metals which we determined through hair analysis. If only I had held off on my haircut a couple days earlier, the doc could have taken off more than the 5 spots she trimmed up to my scalp. Luckily, the samples were small and by choosing ones in the middle of my hair, no one could visibly see them. This test showed normal levels of copper and other metals, but extremely high levels of zinc. In order for many functions to go smoothly in the body, the copper to zinc ratio needs to be approximately 1:8 as they both facilitate some of the previously mentioned biochemistry.[14] In someone with copper toxicity, low plasma zinc levels can actually show up in the hair as high levels of zinc.[15] Essentially, what the hair is indicating is that the zinc is getting displaced from the body and pushed out through the hair. Was that the case for me? I believe so, but sometimes the body will show us things in a different way than we typically would assume via tests. This made me wonder if there was still a missing link. There is also a lot of different types of metal testing, so sometimes it can be difficult to actually receive a true reading. Hair shows a more recent exposure, hence the copper, where as a provoked urinalysis is discussed as a better way to perceive accumulation of metals in tissues internally. Yet, there is controversy around this method.

Regardless, I knew that the toxins had caused a bacterial overgrowth as the white blood cell count was telling in itself. This had to be fixed first in order for anything to else heal since those byproducts and imbalances could affect everything else in the body. My gut was so imbalanced, I could see it in my skin with the never-ending breakouts and dryness, while also feeling it through my crazy cravings.

I allowed my acne to work for me rather than against me though. Using the skin mapping technique, I was able to understand more as to what area of my body was having complications from all the toxins based on which region of my face was troubled. For example, the middle of the cheeks was often related to the inflammation and bacteria of the large intestine. Many ideas online were different in regard to this, so sometimes I had to go with my intuition on what it was communicating.

I felt sick after eating many a days. I knew there was congestion in my liver from filtering all the toxins due to the yellowing in my eyes. Even though I did regular liver flushes, I could feel a rise in pressure about every three weeks as it got tight under my right rib and harder to breathe with this tension in the front of the lungs. The liver enzymes were high on my tests as well, so I had some confirmation on this. For as much as it was congested however, the numbers were only a couple points above normal. This is another point in which I felt our 'normals' were not good enough for indicating overall health.

My next test was an organic acids test. Essentially this test looks at the by-products that are released through urine, indicating where there could be a break in conversion of nutrients. This test can give insight in what you may need more or less of in your diet, if you have a bacterial overgrowth, low neurotransmitters and more. I was low in biotin, which is a B vitamin often associated with skin, nails and hair. There were also signs of bacteria in the amount of harmful acids associated with an overgrowth. The question remained though as to what kind of bacteria. Each strain of bacteria we carry can express itself in a specific way. We could have made a guess as to the types by looking into these by-products, but to truly know for sure, a stool analysis was required.

After that test, I knew which specific bacteria were present versus solely the byproducts. I mentioned my own research in looking up foods that fed these strains, but I also looked up as to what infections or signs of illness these strains could show their ugly selves as in the body. One strain could present itself as urinary tract infections, which explained why I had these so frequently growing up, and I knew my kidneys were not quite what they should be with lack of urgency. The other strain of bacteria showed itself as respiratory infections, or in my case sinus infections, which came up regularly in my life.

The crazy thing about this is that we can all carry different types of bacteria between us, no one person being the same, and anything related to diet or our environment, including stress and emotions, can tip the scales in either a positive or negative way. For some, this is quite the balancing act. The more I have cleansed my body, the more I have also noticed that the minute I do eat something sugary or have an adult beverage, my body responds immediately with bloat, inflammation or congestion. It's my opinion that we tend to get accustomed to overgrowths in our body, and the vengeful bugs will get used to being cohabitants. When we kick their asses to the curb and allow the immune boosting, energizing bugs to take over, it means we are living a healthier lifestyle so suddenly, having a candy bar one day will feel much different than it did when we were living in harmony with the bad guys. The feeling of them trying to overgrow will become more apparent and the symptoms we lived with every day that we clear, will be more noticeable, too.

Parasites are another cohabitant we can test for. I feel we get arrogant as humans thinking that our role on this planet is the most important and we are the only significant life. If we ignore the effects we have on other living creatures and the effects some living creatures have on us, we are missing the bigger picture. Parasites sound disgusting by the name, but this subject is too often overlooked in medicine and it's hard to identify in testing. Most of us have a small number of parasites, whether it be due to walking outside barefoot, owning a pet, or eating under-cooked meat or seafood. Because I detoxed heavily, the toxins fed parasites just as it did bacteria and created more of a problem. Both of these partners in crime love heavy metals! Which is even more of a reason to detox. They will hold onto the metals, allowing the symptoms to also then stick around. Ahhhhhhh!

Luckily in my process I had some divine intervention and

many spiritual experiences. I knew I had support from up in the air, but the idea of 'ask and you shall receive' never became more prominent. I do not believe it matters your faith, when you ask your higher power for assistance and your request is sincere at heart, answers will be provided. In my case, I had a dream parasites were the answer to why I was still not recovering from this. At first, I was thinking 'Really? Is that truly what that dream was?'. As I was perusing the internet in the morning on types of liver stones (you know, a typical kind of morning), I kept being led to videos on parasites. I believe they knew my stubbornness would prevent me from wanting to recognize the truth. After all, I never would have thought something like this would happen to me. I was a clean freak! But that doesn't really matter at the end of the day.

Since I was going off pure faith, I found a few herbs I knew would be effective for nearly all parasites since they obviously were not showing up in testing for me. After taking some of these like wormwood, black walnut hull and clove, I realized my dream was right. I knew because....well...they started to leave. I'll just put it that way. All the chronic pain, fatigue, gastrointestinal issues, acne—heck, I think nearly everything—was related to the nasty chemicals these guys were distributing in my body. I started to feel better nearly immediately, although being extremely fatigued as my body was detoxing an intense amount at once. Feeling blessed in this case is an understatement.

These guys could have been the end of me if they had gotten much worse and I was spared for a reason. They were taking my food, eating my tissues and I could feel them leaving my blood stream even. No wonder I felt as if I had aged 10 years and was malnourished no matter how much I ate. Whole Foods had to love my grocery bill! As I had my blood-work retested, I noticed the most significant changes in relation to treating this were in my iron levels and white blood cells. My previous iron ranges were nearly three times the normal range and my white blood cells were high in some types and low in others. Take this for what you will as we all show up differently. Personally, after seeing how the basics of a healthy life is parallel to bacteria balance and sometimes parasite cleansing, I now recommend this as the first physical detox component in my program for clients so we are not potentially feeding anything as we add more practices with time.

Our belief system breeds these as well, so outside of supplementation, this was another area of intense emotional and energetic healing to take place. Related from anything with body image issues, to victimization, to giving away my power. We are essentially walking bacteria, with it making up 90% of our being.[16] Simple herbs and healing modalities for maintenance in this realm can be important to integrate through our entire lifetime. We put our dogs on heart worm medication, but we don't offer ourselves protection from these basic life forms?

I hear people discuss food allergy testing in a controversial way, with some for it and some against it. If I mention it to someone who has digestive issues and tell them my experiences, "my doctor said it doesn't do much" is a common response. I have done a couple different food allergy tests over the past five years and I agree that it is often hard to decipher if you are in fact allergic to something, or if you eat a specific food so much that it is showing up as an allergy. The first allergy test I experienced, indicated I was allergic to turkey, broccoli, sesame, and wheat. My response was 'Whaaaaaaattttttt?!' Then my allergist explained to me that it could show up strongly if you eat something frequently. Even if that is the case, my body was getting confused as to whether or not these foods were a threat or nourishment.

To determine whether these foods were showing up due to the frequency of my eating them or because of an actual allergy, it was beneficial for me to cut them all out. In doing so, I realized that I did in fact have a wheat allergy. It takes about three weeks to get a food out of your system after eliminating it from your diet, and 72 hours to see if you have an allergy after reintroducing it. If an allergy is more severe, it will typically show up immediately. For some this could be a skin rash, others a cough, stuffiness, maybe trouble breathing. It's different with everyone. For me, I began to have incredibly slow digestion after reintroducing wheat, as well as bloating, sinus irritation and an overall feeling of heaviness in my gut. After reintroducing turkey, sesame (which I ate in the form of hummus) and broccoli, I was fine!

I decided on another allergy test this past year after getting all the other testing back. I had a hunch that with all the stress my body had been under, there was a possibility more foods may show up as reactive in my system. I thought it could give me some information as to what may be feeding any negative gut bacteria, while also allowing me an opportunity to give my immune system a break in what I was able to control during this heavy detoxing. I surely did not want to feed into this anymore than I may already have unknowingly, and I knew my body was going haywire with all these extreme changes happening too quickly.

The cool thing about this test was not only did it test food allergies, it looked at the cooked, raw, and processed forms of some foods. On a food genetic level (because they have genes too), it checked if anything was cross-reactive. This is referring to the fact that sometimes the genes of a food can mimic the genes of another food, causing the body to react the same regardless as to which one you are eating. For instance, sesame actually has a gene in it similar to wheat, so when the body is breaking down food, it can question whether or not it needs to protect itself against sesame in someone like myself that has a wheat allergy. Although I did not have any new severe allergies show up in this test, it did reconfirm how important it is to mix up my diet since so many foods I had been eating frequently appeared as sensitivities again. If we eat the same things over and over, it throws the body off and confuses it as to why this is a reoccurring particle entering the body. For someone like me who had to avoid sulfurs, wheat, and dairy, along with my own choice in avoiding corn, trying to food prep for the week while mixing in more variety to what I eat was difficult. I tried to look at it as an opportunity to be creative, rather than a challenge that was limiting me.

I used to be shy in restaurants to ask for substitutions or request something be cooked in olive oil rather than butter, but not anymore! My health has become too much of a priority to worry about whether the kitchen is rolling their eyes. Although the movie *Waiting* replays in my head from time to time, I try to imagine that was an exaggeration of what truly goes down behind the scenes. The restaurants that do understand, are my go tos and appreciate my repeat business no matter the dietary guidelines.

Genetics! I never had an opportunity to investigate my genes until I had to this year. My next analysis was "23 and Me," which is a company often advertised for genetic testing. It allows people a chance to see what diseases they may be prone to, now or in the future, based on their family history and if they themselves are carriers. It can also determine anything from your dominant muscle fiber type to improve workouts, what your eye color might be, and your sensitivity in smell. With everything that was going on in my body, the chemistry was becoming more important to me personally to make sure there was no damage done from toxins. I was also in the "go big or go home" mindset at this point when it came to tests. I felt we looked at every-thing else, and the opportunity presented itself so let's keep on chuggin' along!

There are a couple different websites you can pay to import your genetic data to further the analysis from "23 and Me", so you can get an actual print-out of the genes you carry, rather than the information regarding how they are expressed, such as eye color. This allowed my doctor to see how my DNA code effected my health overall, and if there were any genes that might even be absent. She also mapped out the pathways in which these genes feed into one another. I was able to see that the CBS gene mutated, which meant my body was not removing those sulfurs properly in one of the liver detox pathways. It also indicated I was not producing enough of an important antioxidant that cleans the cells, called glutathione. I found some information that led me to understand this genetic mutation could also exhaust other genes, in particular one that helps in serotonin and melatonin production. I began to look at my supplement regimen again and make sure I was taking the appropriate options that would support both of these genes so neither were overburdened, or another mutation was encouraged.

As you can tell, the genetics piece of this puzzle can be complicated and if you decide to learn more on your own outside of what you are told, the information can be outstanding and dense at the same time. I almost felt as if I was going back to school for my own doctorate as I found myself continuously intrigued and engulfed in article after article. The black hole of the world wide web.

Regular blood testing continued as I wanted to make sure we were seeing improvements. Although, my bloodwork still isn't perfect, I am feeling better and more like the Amanda I am familiar with. Sometimes the body needs time to adjust. I detoxed so hard at once, that it screamed at me and in order to please it, I had to do everything in my power of supplementing, therapies, and testing to keep it happy. When our bodies get used to functioning in a specific way with toxins, similarly to the bacteria imbalance, it can easily get thrown off when we make an extreme change. This is why it is so important to detox slowly. I may have learned a tremendous amount in my own process of extreme detox, but my experience from this will hopefully teach others and support them in doing it in a way that will not have as much of a life-threatening effect.

Out of all the tests I took, I felt that besides the standard blood test, the stool analysis and the gene testing were the most useful tests. It's easy to assume we all have a dysbiosis of some kind, knowing what the bacteria strains are can provide you with important information in what foods will support us, and what antimicrobials, antibacterial, and or antifungals will help to balance it out.

YOUR DETOX

All Kinds of Kinds

Know your normals! If you go to the doctor for your yearly physicals, take an active role and actually go into that portal and look at your blood work. Keep copies of these each year and store them in a file. Like I mentioned, many normal lab ranges are taken from a sample group, and there are only so many variables. Much is left to the unknown. So the best way to know what's normal in your body? Be your own data collector. This doesn't mean you have to spend hours like I did in going through my own analyses, but if you have anything change significantly, you can refer to your baseline. Just compare numbers as you get your check-ups to the previous year and be aware if numbers go up or down in a drastic way. Regardless if they are shown as being abnormal or not.

Although stool testing was helpful, jump down to the next chapter on supplementation and my perspective on bacteria and parasites. We can definitely pay to test, but there is a lot being discovered to this day when it comes to these topics. Many herbs are multi-faceted and can take care of these guys, regardless as to whether we have "discovered" them in our results. As long as there are no contraindications to medications or health concerns, these herbs should be harmless. As with anything, you can see how your body responds and take it from there with some professional guidance.

Designer 'Genes'

My overall favorite test was genetic testing. Genes can change expression with emotional, environmental, and dietary influences, which is often referred to as epigenetics. Most negative gene expressions however can be reversed, and some studies are showing actual gene mutations causing disease, can often be controlled through diet and lifestyle as well.[17] Analyzing the results through testing is empowering as it gives insight not only on how the genes are effected and what you might be a carrier of, but if you are able to see a map of the genes together, you can better understand how they feed into each other. This mapping can be a determinant of what the root of a health problem could be.

After utilizing the "23 and Me "site, along with downloading and mapping the metabolic cycles of these genes with my doctor, we were able to see where the breaks were in the systems of my body. By learning how the negative effects of some genes cascaded to others and inhibited there function, I was able to understand what I could do to support those genes while healing the mutations. Looking at the health of the physical body in terms of nutrition, mindset and emotional practices, are what we can personally control to improve these outcomes. Changing the neural pathways as mentioned when it comes to self-care practices and energy healing, can change the whole functionality of the body as everything is controlled by the nervous system.

Stand Up

Through testing and understanding the numerous angles we can peer at our health, but there's still only so much analytical data we can look at on the outside without truly knowing what's going on inside of us. So many tiny chemical exchanges are happening second to second, minute to minute. There were days that I woke up and ran to get my blood test early in the morning before I ate, after not sleeping well a few nights in a row. Sometimes this threw off my glucose and other metabolic measurements. Testing is a wonderful tool and provides so much insight, but similarly to how different diet fads give us a start in understanding what makes our bodies feel better, there's a level of intuition we need to reveal what our bodies require. So much is left undiscovered when it comes to the biology of the body even, so again we need to assume that testing is not the end all be all, but a tool for guidance. Our bodies are so intelligent, and it becomes easy to forget that they have our best interest at heart.

Physicians are people we entrust with our lives as to what will be beneficial when they analyze our level of health and wellness. The problem I found was that I was taking no action in understanding what we were testing for and why, until I saw something in red. Detoxification has taught me to reconnect with my body and take an active role in advocating for my own health, even if it's simply knowing the right questions to ask. When we rely too much on one person to do all the work, not to mention a person who also has a life and stressors of their own personal accord, we can lose a sense of ourselves. It's not to say that you cannot trust, but that just like any everyday relationship, working together and communicating produces the best outcomes. In the current medical system outside of functional, integrative, or naturopathy practices, the body is typically treated as parts (you go to your gynecologist if you're a woman to examine your female organs, your orthopedist when you have an issue with your bones and muscles, and your endocrinologist when you have diabetes or thyroid issues, for instance) and not a whole. Everything works together, and when that's happening properly, detoxification will come naturally. Thus, the health we decide to implement in our lives will prevent further accumulation of toxins.

SUMMARY

So how can we get started in approaching our personalized testing? Labtestsonline.com is an excellent resource if you have questions on bloodwork. This is a great way to get started in understanding what basic measurements are taken and what they mean. The more we understand and take interest in the quality of our bodies, the more educated questions we can ask. Reflect on how you want to utilize your time here, whether it be beneficial to do research on your own, or ask another professional to assist you. Getting another perspective can bring attention to ideas we may be unaware of in communicating our health. If we can work with our physicians, rather than tasking them to make all the calls, I believe we could have more productive outcomes, not to mention a more functional relationship.

CHAPTER 7: THE ALTERNATIVES

After trying to become more holistic over the past few years prior to toxicity, I remained incredibly headstrong in maintaining this mission throughout my detox and recovery. I did feel seemingly lost at times, and there was a moment I decided to take an antibiotic due to severe pain and fever from a bacterial infection. Outside of this, I tried every alternative therapy and supplement that would help my process to avoid additional damage from chemicals. It can cost a lot of money to go the holistic route, but it's my hope that in explaining some of my experience and how I apply it to my program as a Health Coach and Energy Healer, I can guide you in budgeting for alternative therapies and supplements if you wish to test them out, too. Depending on your health situation, you might be able to expedite the healing process by adding these to your tool box.

MY DETOX

My first experience in trying to correct my health was through supplementation. I feel that addressing the body in testing, stress, and other areas should come first before blindly taking supplements without indicators as to why or what would be helpful. When I first started feeling sick, I was so clueless as to how to approach this that I decided to become my own experiment and trial and error supplements. Since it took me a few months to find a doctor to identify heavy metals as the source of my toxicity, I was attempting to do anything I could on my own to get through the days. I do not recommend this for you, but for me it was the only thing that made sense at the time. I started off by supplementing with B vitamins, magnesium, probiotics, a multivitamin, and fish oil as I could tell both my nervous system and gut health were off. Even though these provided some relief, I was still not myself and the fatigue and muscle pain were a huge frustration.

As I completed the multiple tests mentioned in chapter seven, we adjusted my supplement regimen as things improved overtime and new information showed up test to test. I noticed my intuition kick in when it came to supplements too, and again I overlooked it, not understanding why. I have a morning, noon and evening pill box for each day of the week, and I would prep every Sunday because frankly, there were too many supplement containers to unscrew every morning. As I would prepare my supplements, there were times when I would question my needs for taking what seemed to be a ridiculous amount. I wanted to make sure I wasn't taking anything more than I needed, and also as the capsules were adding up, the stress on my digestion and body as a whole was counterproductive. With so much in the mix, how did I know my body was truly able to absorb all of it? Especially with the body's tendency to pick and choose what vitamins and minerals it will absorb whether you intend to take them all in. With my liver under enough pressure to rid me of chemicals, the last thing I wanted to do was add more responsibilities to its list. My digestive tract needed to concentrate on healing, and although some supplements were to help with that, the state of my body needed to be considered as to whether it had the energy for all of the above. There were also times I knew a supplement would be good for me, and other times when I could not even look at the bottle as it repulsed me. If I questioned this feeling, I might look it up and double check what it was doing for me on a biological level. In trying to understand this feeling, it would throw me for a loop. Why was I having this response and was it important? Was it simply that there were too many tablets I was taking, or did it indicate something else?

Turns out I was on a lot of Sulfur based supplements. The irony is that the supplements I often questioned contained them. Occasionally I instinctually knew to increase or decrease my zinc, too. This was no accident in adjusting my regimen either, indicating I was not getting enough in my diet and I still had too much copper or other toxins interrupting different functions. Since the ratio to copper and zinc needed to be considered, I could tell when I cut out zinc that my progress seemed to decline some. This happened many other times in regard to other supplements as I continued to heal. I never would have imagined my body having an intuition so intense, that it could pick up on specific supplements being good or bad for me, too little or too much. I would not recommend playing with your supplements in this way until you speak with a physician and learn this response as you acclimate. It took me a lot of research and time in developing this relationship with myself, but the law of attraction applies to a lot more than just the Tinder app. Even though we are born with intuitive tools, toxins, along with a world created of distractions from the relationship to ourselves, can prevent us from tapping into what the body is asking for and how to interpret this.

As far as supplements go, I could give you 50 pages of the ones I tried, why I tried them, the benefits I saw and the effects they had on my body. I personally took up to 60 tablets a day at times. Looking back, regardless as to how much these were keeping me moving and preventing infections, I don't encourage this. For someone detoxifying in a slower more physically efficient manner, you should not have to spend or consume nearly as much, and often the cheapest healthful solutions can make the biggest difference.

One of those amazingly cost-efficient solutions would be a clove of garlic. I noticed a big response in my body by simply eating a clove of garlic here and there. Although it has a lot of Sulfur and I did have to avoid it for a while, garlic has a ton of health benefits, including being a natural antimicrobial, antibacterial, and antifungal. Local honey, especially Manuka honey, acts the same and you can even mix these with garlic to lighten the punch of chewing garlic. Bacteria, like the ever-popular H. Pylori, have been linked to stomach ulcers, and Manuka honey has been mentioned as an aid in repairing them. I use manuka honey topically for burns or cuts due to its healing properties, and on my face as well to kill acne related bacteria, while improving scarring. Apply it for 15 minutes as a face mask to kill bacteria and aid in healing the skin. The only hazard in this is to make sure you are careful with the types of bacteria, because too much honey can have the reverse affect whether you are using it topically or ingesting it.[18]

Bentonite clay was another supplement I would take on occasion with a tablespoon in some warm water to be sure it mixed nicely. Along with removing most other things in the body, it helps in detoxing heavy metals. Most bentonite clays are marked whether or not they are food grade. Activated charcoal can support the same while alkalizing the body and keeping down inflammation. They also act as great face masks when left on for 20 minutes! Both bentonite and charcoal will pull anything out of anywhere you apply it. We are referring to the gut and skin mostly, for those of you with your minds in the gutter. When taking either of these, it is advised to use them 90 minutes before or after any eating or supplementation. Although they are pulling out the bad, they can also prevent your body from absorbing nutrition from foods and other factors.[19]

I loved utilizing herbs in my healthscapade because of their simplicity and price point. Some parsley and cilantro steeped in hot water with my teas were a great way to support detox as cilantro removes metals, and parsley can cleanse the kidneys. Keeping the detox pathways supported is key in making sure you are actually removing them from the body versus recirculating them. Sage, thyme and rosemary are also potent antibacterial and antimicrobials.[20]

The list of therapies is endless and can be overwhelming in learning where to begin. One thing I found to be incredibly important as I journeyed through the land of toxins was keeping an open mind to any and all practices that were suggested. I was already on more supplements than I could count on my fingers and toes, and I knew this was unrealistic long-term. I wanted to do the best I could to get rid of all this toxic build-up, but what else was a girl to do? With my doctor offering tons of alternate ways to detox the body, I was able to try some things in office. I began with infrared sauna, tested the hyperbaric chamber, Rife therapy, ST-8—you name it, I was on it.

YOUR DETOX

Sometimes finding out what supports your body is what we would least suspect, because typically we are focused on processing with our head and not our heart. When you feel a resistance to trying something new, the key to intuition is asking yourself why. Is it your gut telling you it won't work, or are you being resistant to change? If it's not standard to what we are assumed to believe is the "right way," that's okay, but is it another box we need to break out of? That thought process applies to this situation as well. It's like trying on clothes at the mall: you might hate a certain shirt on the rack, but when you give it a chance and try it on, it's the one thing you end up buying. With everything I have done, I will give you the run down on my favorites, even some I expected to dislike but were most effective as I continued to tap into that intuition.

Supplements

What's the first priority in your physical health? Have you done regular testing to offer any evidence as to where you are lacking in diet or what you may not be absorbing from food? At the end of the day, supplements can be just as much of a band-aid as prescriptions, even though they may take on more of a natural form. If we are solely relying on something to make us feel better yet can never come off it, we are not getting to the root of the problem. The blood recycles itself every 90 days, so many times, you should see a major difference in that time-frame, depending on the severity of symptoms you are experiencing, or how they are interconnected. Most of us have some sort of compromised digestion, so making sure we are getting the most out of our food is important.

National Geographic may portray the symbiotic nature of this planet in a more desirable way, but just because we are not living in the Sahara dessert, doesn't mean we are void of this. Back to bacteria and parasites! These basic forms of life of bacteria and parasites are passed through the placenta as well, so it's no longer our health problems, it's our future generations to come. I bring this up again because it is so entirely important in the big picture on so many levels. Incorporating supplementation to support this is much needed and will aid in the absorption of food overtime, mentioned above. The byproducts produced by these guys can cause anything from autoimmune diseases, to neurological disorders, to digestive issues, to cancer and other terminal illnesses.[21]

I believe if we were to address these two components alone, we would have a healthier nation both physically and mentally. After a full-on consistent cleanse, we benefit from a maintenance dose of these herbs on a weekly basis. Even if a client does not 'think' they have it, I still recommend considering it. Our bodies become acclimated and adapt to even the negative cycles, or in this case cohabitants, for survival purposes. Toxins released in the body during future detox practices feeds this, which I learned the hard way. Before integrating additional detox methods, it's important to clear this component so we can set ourselves up for success and less inhibitions to our process. Don't wait until symptoms are too difficult to address to rule this out.

The absolute necessary ingredients you should look for in purchasing a supplement or cleanse of this kind (because there are so many for purchase these days) are black walnut hull, wormwood, and clove.[22] Additional beneficial ingredients are diatomaceous earth, mimosa pudica, garlic, and most other herbs are helpful, too. A few controversial methods include hydrogen peroxide therapy where you dilute a 35% food grade version in water, turpentine (100% pure gum spirits-not the store-bought paint stripper), and MMS (Miracle Mineral Solution). These I feel people need to decide for themselves or with their doctor since there are not many studies published on them. They are hard on the body and you can have some pretty extreme die off symptoms because if your body is burdened, it will kill them off almost more quickly than your body can handle. I made the decision to try this because I was unable to tell how bad it had gotten, and I was mentally in a state of emergency. I soon found out after taking them that it was pretty severe. However, it worked in my own body so I believe if you are out of solutions and need to widen the variety, it's worth looking in to. Plus, certain solutions claim to stay active in the body longer, hence getting where we need them to go. Too many supplements can oxidize fairly quickly after taken, so we want to approach not only the quality and source, but activity level and distribution.

Integrity in the digestive lining, along with regularity and consistency is always a priority. If after the bacteria cleanse you still feel any digestive distress, we would move forward in addressing this. Of course, it depends on the individual and the particular form of distress, but many of us have either consti-pation or diarrhea. For the first, I would recommend herbal teas (which is always my first choice due to price and being more available to the body as a liquid) or supplements that increase regularity while still supporting the mucosal lining (the intestinal tract has mucosal secretions to keep things moving like a well-oiled machine, or a line at Marshall's department stores for us fashion seekers). My top choices in supporting the belly through all of this is licorice, aloe, marshmallow, and senna. There are many herbal blends out there and they can also have multiple benefits. These four will be great additions if you purchase a blend as they soothe and support that intestinal lining, while acting as antibacterials and gentle laxatives.[23] I prefer taking supplements for this purpose in the evening before bed if they do not already recommend it, so they can stay in the digestive tract a little longer. We eliminate more successfully in the morning, as it's our body's natural tendency anyway.

Since we are assuming these digestive complications are still around after a bacterial cleanse, chances are we have a depletion of the good guys and we need to replenish them. Starting with some prebiotic fibers is typically better to recreate our personal bacteria profile, so eating a green banana, oats, adding psyllium husks or chia to the diet can assist with this when coming from a food source perspective. You can also purchase prebiotic fibers in a tablet form, too. For those of us that have been on dozens of antibiotics (holla), we may need a little oomph from the pros.

If the digestive tract is moving along Taylor swiftly, then I look at how we can support the liver. Similarly to bacteria, if we do not make sure the body is eliminating efficiently and then go on to detox other areas, we are basically causing them to recirculate. So if they are staying in the body, while also giving us side effects, we are the source of our own demise. The liver being supportive of so many chemical reactions and energetic exchanges needs some TLC regularly. Again, I think herbal teas are great for this, and one of my favorites called "Everyday Detox" has a combination of other herbs and natural sources to support more than just the liver. Looking for a boost from sources such as milk thistle, dandelion, burdock and chicory help to increase the function and health of the liver.[24] Also eating liver once a week (because it's so high in copper that's all you'd require) or taking liver supplements that have been sourced from organic farm-raised cows is an option. If we eat liver or take a supplement of the source (really in regard to any organ for that matter), we are introducing nearly identically composed tissues, that when broken down in our body, help to assist in restoration of our own organs. Stay focused on the repair and support.

More is not always better when it comes to supplements either. Many times, we think we should load up on everything to cover our ground, but the body breaks all of this down and adjusts to what's entering just like it would foods. This can overwhelm our stomach in adjusting acidity, pancreatic enzymes, and the liver and gallbladder come into play as well. It's best to choose a few supplements or symptoms to address first, and slowly add supplements to the routine. Keep a journal by your side or a rolling note in your phone. If you notice any discomfort throughout the day, then you can look at what you changed in your routine versus the timing of this side effect. Also, some supplements go together, while some supplements act as antagonists. For example, vitamin E and selenium should always be taken together, but if you take too much zinc, it could imbalance your copper. It also depends on what you eat them with. For example, fat soluble vitamins like A, D, E and K, are best absorbed while being taken with a meal consisting of some fat. Try to be strategic if you can so your supplements are not competing, and they are gaining optimal absorption.

Alternative Therapies
When it comes to choosing alternative therapies, first decide on your budget. The ones I have tried can range anywhere from $25 to $150. As we discuss them, I will rate these therapies monetarily with a $-$$$ next to the name in reference to those price ranges. Would you be interested in this once a month? Per week? Decide on the frequency as well based on the amount of time you have. Many of them can take up to 90 minutes, so for most of us making time in a busy schedule has to be well thought out.

Infrared Sauna $
One of my favorite therapies is infrared sauna, which is different than a regular sauna we might associate with. Our body should naturally sweat, but sometimes toxins can build-up and prevent this function by accumulating in the tissues. For me, unless I was doing an intense hot yoga class, or running myself into the ground via athletic conditioning, I "glistened" as we ladies like to say, instead of really sweating. The idea of introducing heat to the body is that our body has to work to cool itself, so in trying to maintain that balance our heart rate increases and metabolically we work harder, which leads to burning calories. Because of the types of light waves you are receiving from the infrared, you are able to pull out more toxins and therefore take

some of the pressure off of your immune system that might be trying to intensely rid your body of them on its own. This in turn gives you energy in other areas of your body, since you've freed yourself of stress in the form of toxic build-up.[25]

There's also a theory that niacin used in conjunction with an infrared sauna will further the effects. Niacin is B3 and it helps to vasodilate or increase the size of your red blood cells. Oxygen itself is a natural cleanser and binds to toxins for removal. The Niacin allows the blood cells to take in more oxygen and improve its distribution, removing more from the tissues deeper in the body surrounding our organs. So, if we can increase the flow of oxygen to these areas of the body, more toxins will be removed by the blood, and then being in the sauna, you sweat them out preventing re-accumulation.[26] Many articles out there will offer up their opinions on how much Niacin you should take for this. Again, always check with your doctor and see what their recommendation is. For me, about 100mg was enough and anything more than that was a little overwhelming for my body. That could be because of its sensitive disposition at the time, but regardless I stopped there and did not push myself to increase the dosage.

Acupuncture $$

Another favorite for me is Acupuncture. As a Chinese Medicine practice, Acupuncture is thought to help in the flow of energy channels throughout the body. When these channels or "meridian" lines are stimulated through the pressure of tiny needles, the energy can flow freely and improve health conditions that might be the result of disrupted energy. In Western medicine, there are multiple theories on how this works, but consistently it's believed to be exciting the nervous system somehow to release hormones or possibly growth factors, which tend to the body's healing and regulate it.[27]

Everyone is treated based on what ails them. For instance, if you are not breaking down fats properly and you know it has to do with your gallbladder, the acupuncturist would focus on the gallbladder meridian line. I've come in with only symptoms before as well, and with my practitioner's help we decided what might be the causation and treated it accordingly. I've specifically used acupuncture to treat my nervous system and gut motility with great results. It can depend on the reason for treatment, but sometimes consecutive treatments are needed until the body starts to adapt on its own. This was one therapy I was skeptical about, as the idea of energy healing was new to me. With my brain trained by our current medical system, I was curious as to what meridian lines are and why this would potentially heal me. Keeping an open mind however, my body showed me that it was responding well to energy healing so I gave it what it needed.

Reiki and Shamanic Healing $$

In keeping with the energy healing theme, my next go around in that arena was Reiki and a Shamanic session. I had Reiki brought up to me a few times. Finally, I said, "Okay universe, I hear you!" With being slightly skeptical with Acupuncture, you can imagine how skeptical I was with Reiki. Only knowing at the time that it helped in opening chakras seemed far out to me, but when you are feeling bad and keep asking for guidance, you'll do anything you can and listen to the signs that present themselves.

I would have emptied my bank account if it meant my quality of life returned.

Now that I am a believer, I can better explain that the idea behind Reiki is healing the body through adjusting your chakras. Chakras are part of the energetic field of our body, which align front-facing 3-4 inches in front of us, then connecting to the spinal cord. We have seven main bodily chakras and energy healers that utilize them such as Reiki, Shamanic and other practitioners, make sure they are aligned in speed and direction. They are not only related to physical health, but emotional health. This modality is harder to prove because energy is difficult to measure and be seen by the eye. It's more less based on personal experience and testimonies, however many I have seen to be positive. You can also cleanse the chakras of heavy energy and traumas.

I mentioned earlier that resentment and anger can be stored in the liver and gallbladder. My first treatment in Reiki brought this to my attention as well, without me even saying much. The Reiki practitioner could feel the heat coming from that area and in using the energy from her hands, she was able to adjust the flow of energy which allowed my body to properly detox this. This was the most rapid healing experience I ever had. Let's just say my body started releasing toxins in some unexpected ways from adjusting the chakras…anything from increased bathroom breaks, wild dreams to reconcile the past, even boils from released anger. I truly began to understand what drudged up emotions of the past could be preventing my healing. After getting treated a couple of times, I began to become more sensitive to this energy flow in my body, and I could tell when it was off. I would get irritable or feel mentally stuck. After another session, I may have some 'releasing' symptoms, but typically after a day or two I would start to feel amazing. The more I went, the less downtime I had after, eventually becoming energized by it.

I had a similar experience with my Shamanic sessions when it came to realigning and cleansing chakras. We also dug into cutting what is called 'energetic chords' that we can spiritually attach to each other, as well as returning soul pieces and fragments that we can give away. Some of the relationships that I had encountered in the past, were still lingering due to the energetic exchanges such as these between myself and the people involved. Letting go of the past had a whole new meaning for me after this. I also completed some ancestral healing, as traumas experienced by family can be genetically passed on since it shifts the DNA. I could feel an immediate release as I worked on these pieces, and there was a level of feeling whole within myself that felt foreign to me. Even though the idea of past lives can often be associated with specific religions, I have seen some of mine in visions and healing these traumas as well added to my improved physical state. I no longer feel that we need to divide this idea into a societal belief system, however this personalized experience is not meant to encourage specific beliefs itself. To each their own.

These are therapies that I will continue to do today as it has not only helped me physically, but in addressing some of the old emotions that needed to go, I have been able to tackle some demons that I didn't even know existed. Sometimes we bury things so deeply, we have trouble even recalling what we need to let go of to move forward. Some great memories I had repressed as well flooded back, and there were days when I was laughing and crying in the same 24 hours. Sometimes to get through pain we purposefully try to avoid confronting the bad situations by forgetting, but the good can also get shoved away in the process. Therefore, I feel it's important to acknowledge all emotions and productively confront them because we wouldn't be fair to ourselves or our bodies by avoiding them, as they are a catalyst in moving forward and learning how we want to grow. The good memories should always be along for the ride, too.

Cryotherapy and Ice Baths $$
Who wants to sit in an ice bath for 10 minutes? Not me! I resorted to freezing my skin for 3 minutes instead. Exposure to extreme cold such as the -200 degrees (or colder) Fahrenheit in a Cryotherapy chamber has been shown to provide benefits by stimulating the nervous system, and there have been studies showing it assisted in healing injuries of athletes. Although few strong studies out there make it somewhat controversial, like many alternate therapies, I had to decide for myself.

I noticed a difference in energy levels, digestion, and reversing muscle fatigue at least for a short period of time. Due to the body's fight or flight response, your brain chemistry adapts as blood flow constricts. This affects many of our biological systems outside of the nervous system-since it controls everything-such as the endocrine system, digestion, immune response, metabolism, and so on. Your body composition can play a role on this as well, because adipose or 'fatty' tissue can prevent the facilitation of cold through the air as its purpose is to insulate, therefore also prevent any possible healing effects of cryotherapy. Ice baths have actually been shown to be more effective if you decide

AMANDA GABBERT

to go that route, as ice has a more advantageous heat transfer capability, meaning it will be successful in removing heat from the body via a solid rather than air and water. Considering your needs, tolerance and body fat percentage, you have plenty of cool options.[28]

Theta Healing $$
Theta healing is another consistent energetic therapy I integrate into my routine. In general, we all have a belief system, right? We've created this whether it was beliefs we absorbed from exposure to others, or ideas we decided to believe based on experiences. These beliefs can have a lot to do with how we perceive the world around us, but that is also an indication of what we think about ourselves. If beliefs block us from becoming abundantly happy in what we want out of life, then we have to get rid of them. Just like Reiki, sometimes the beliefs require discovery by someone else because we bury the experiences to cope. There is also our own level of bias that can prevent us from seeing the bigger picture.

In Theta Healing, a practitioner is able to spiritually tap into your being and assist you in muscle testing for beliefs that have developed on the soul level, effecting the other energetic layers of the body. They can also look through their third eye and energetically see any blockages in your body. You tap into your intuition to start identifying the inner dialogue. Let's use the belief "money is stressful," for instance. This is very topical and something that is easy for us to say as the client, because it's on our mind all the time. The practitioner then helps us to get to the root belief that this is coming from. Some can be as simple

107

as asking the universe or your higher divine to remove the belief and that's that. Others, like this one for example, can have many layers, like an onion. Let's say the practitioner continues to ask questions in regard to the stress of money. After many questions, you get down to "I'm worthless." Although money being stressful is a component, the basis of this belief that was also feeding many other beliefs, was "I am worthless." Kind of like an upside-down food pyramid with one serving of worthlessness and 12 servings of other frustrations and pain, money incorporated.

Getting to the root of beliefs can relieve a lot of emotions and change our day to day interactions as we begin to value ourselves more and start attracting better experiences. In turn, the physical effects in the body or symptoms these beliefs co-created will also begin to clear. Alongside removing beliefs, we also did a lot of inner child healing, chord cutting, returning of soul pieces, and a number of other modalities in releasing spiritual attachments and traumas from this life and previous lives. Wowza! If only I could have told my soul to stop giving itself away too 20 years ago.

IV Therapy $$$
IV therapy has become a popular way to add a higher dose of vitamins, minerals and nutrients straight to the blood stream, thus bypassing the gut. If we are what we absorb, many of us cannot entirely assimilate what we need from our encapsulated supplements and food. This is a great way to get a boost. Because you are also getting incredibly hydrated, be sure to let the clinic know when you start to feel bloated or have that "full" feeling. My stature is fairly small, so although the office I went to offered two IV bags, I could only handle one. You will feel this for the

remainder of the day or into the next, depending on the time you received it, but it's water weight so it will slowly filter out of the body.

Most places will categorize the treatments whether they're focused on energy, detox, post-exercise, post-hangover... the list goes on. The cost for me was about $125, and the effects are very temporary. I would say it's great if you are in a dire situation or really feeling low. If you try this and it really resonates in your body, go as often as your budget allows! Always be careful about taking in an extensive number of vitamins that your body may be better off without though. Most excess B vitamins will pass right through you; however, some excess vitamins and minerals can accumulate in tissues if you are taking too much over long periods of time.

Hyperbaric $$$

Hyperbaric chambers are used by a lot of athletes, who have helped to create its popularity. This one would cost me about $150 a session and if you purchase packages you typically get a better deal. It's another therapy that the consistency is important with if you have a specific ailment. Due to the decreasing availability of oxygen to us in our environment and thinning atmosphere, this pressurized chamber induces oxygen into the body from the outside through the skin. With oxygen having the ability to kill anything abnormal in the body and to increase healing, you can see how this is a solution for nearly everything.[29] If you have the bucks, do it a few times a week until you feel the healing in your body. If you are looking to have an extra boost, one session may do you some good. It's more of a go big or go home when it comes to extreme healing. Cost-wise, magnesium oxide at home may help if you prefer the oxygen route via supplementation, even if it is a minute amount in comparison.

Although there are a TON of therapies that you could choose to invest in, there are also a lot of options to take care of yourself at home.

At Home Therapies

Sound therapy is music created to promote healing based on specific energetic vibrations produced by the sounds themselves. Sound silly? How many of you out there have a favorite song that lifts your spirits on a bad day? It's the same thing, just in a different light. Music creates feeling and emotion which is energy, and we feel this all the way down to the carbon molecules that make us. You can pay for this if you'd like to find someone to cater this art specifically to you, however with all the money going out on other alternate routes, I found some great sound bites on YouTube. Just search whatever your concern is next to the word "binaural beats." For instance, I entered "digestive healing binaural beats" one day and an hour-long video appeared. Because these music compositions are mostly instrumental, they are excellent to have on in the background at work, while you're doing chores, etc. They're peaceful and can help in focus as well.

To remove toxins via your mouth, there are techniques such as oil pulling where you swish coconut oil around in your mouth for 20 minutes. You could also try tongue scraping. Using a tongue scraping tool with a few strokes in the morning and evening, scrapes the bacteria off your tongue, adding to your tooth-brushing routine. Personally, I have a hard time fitting the oil pulling in, but I do tongue scrape on occasion. This is another little guy in comparison to other therapies, but some people may prefer to do a bunch of little things on their own than pay for multiple large options.

Another favorite of mine is dry brushing. Dry brushing uses a dry bath brush to rub your skin in the direction of your lymphatic system to remove toxins and get your blood flowing. There is a lot of contradiction out there on researching this, but the increased blood flow acts similarly as a brisk walk would in increasing blood flow, hence oxygen as well. I prefer this in the morning since it can feel very invigorating and energizing to start the day. It also exfoliates your skin. I love doing this on the days that I don't exercise in the morning so I am getting similar benefits while allowing my body some rest. Emotionally, physical touch is important to our well-being and nurturing ourselves in this way is just as nurturing as it is coming from someone else. Plus, it can be considered meditative in the sense that it is offering time to connect with your body and mind. When you pick out a brush, harder bristles are not better. You need a light touch to do the job, so pick soft or medium bristles and usually you can easily find a round natural fiber brush with a handle for easy grip. Looking up dry brushing videos is the best way to make sure you are doing it correctly. It's important to go in a specific direction with the brush so you are properly encouraging the lymph flow. In general, most would describe it as brushing towards the heart. Massages are great as well for the lymph, along with the overall bodywork.

The Neti pot, also known as a sinus rinse, is an excellent way to cleanse the sinus cavity. We breathe in particles all day long and there's so much that gets kicked up into our system, whether it be exhaust from cars, or pollutants from factories. I have some outdoor allergies as well and I love doing this to make sure I don't have pollen residue where it can be most irritating. If I start to get stuffy regularly or feel a possible sinus infection coming on, I will do this a few times a day. Especially at night as the cool air encourages the pollen to sink in the atmosphere, making it more readily available to our noses and easily carried inside from our clothes and hair. If you are in the same boat with allergies, showering at night is also good, so you prevent the pollination of your bedding. Be sure you are using purified water, or boiling tap water and then allowing it to cool prior. Clean water in this at home gem is top priority!

Drum roll please…last but not least, the ultimate at home, 10 on a scale of 10 grossness, the coffee enema. When this was suggested to me, well, I blocked out every word that came out of my doctor's mouth after the initial words of "coffee enema." Then I decided "what the heck?" in my desperateness to feel like Amanda again. I mean, there's a book called *Everybody Poops* that we are introduced to as toddlers, so as an adult I should be able to handle this. With the colon being the first line of detox-ification, I needed to assist it in rectifying (see what I did there) the situation. I purchased a silicone enema, as this material is not going to pass added chemicals like containers made from plastic. I already brewed coffee in the morning, so adding a little more to the pot wasn't difficult. Set aside a cup and let it cool. The purpose of the enema is not simply to shoot coffee in the opposite direction that we typically associate it with.

The colon runs alongside what's called the portal vein. The

portal vein runs to the liver, so not only are you washing out any pockets of the colon and stimulating its motility, you are also encouraging liver function. I briefly mentioned glutathione earlier being an antioxidant that cleanses cells, and it's produced by the liver. With the liver being stimulated by the portal vein, it's now also increasing production of glutathione.[30] The thought process of coffee compared to the way traditional saline enemas work, is that the coffee encourages more blood flow because caffeine is a stimulant. Therefore, in proximity to the portal vein, and in increasing the blood flow, it can effectively care for the liver, whereas saline is simply to cleanse and hydrate the colon.

The topic of enemas can be controversial. Some people say they can be very depleting, while others will make claims they saved their lives. There are not many studies on these, however by trying it I was able to see for myself. It helped quite a bit and when I was initially very sick, I did them a lot because the improvement was noticeable. I felt energized by them and I needed all the energy I could get. Let's just say, coffee was incredibly hard to keep in the house. After I detoxed more, I felt the need to do these less and less. On the other end of the process (also another spot for joke insertion), I began to feel a little more depleted by them. This might be in conjunction with my liver detoxification being inhibited with the gene mutation, but there's no real way to determine this.

SUMMARY

When it comes to choosing what alternative therapies work for you, sometimes you need to gauge how you feel in doing so and go with your gut. That ever impressive intuition will work its magic again. The other piece to trying new things is as we are detoxing, sometimes you can feel sick depending on what kinds of therapies you do since you are encouraging removal of toxins. I would check with your practitioner if you have one you work with on all remedies and make sure any post-detox symptoms you have are normal, while also being sure there are no contra-indications to medications or potential side effects based on your health history.

We all respond differently to things but gauging our bodies' response is important when we are releasing things that shouldn't be there. If anything, this is evident in my experience that when an intense 'healing crisis' does come about, see if there is a way you can still detox while taking it down a notch to avoid adding to the physical load. We never want to add to the potential of causing trauma in a different way.

CHAPTER 8: WHY THE DAMN DETOX?

MY WHY

I had gotten to a point in my life that required a lot of reflection. Bad relationships, negative body image, constant comparison. I never spoke my true voice, and this hurt me physically more than anything. I lost who I was while I became focused on making other people happy. I had negative beliefs based on my experiences that allowed fear to run my life, and when I began to experience illness in such a way it was life threatening, I asked myself, "If today were my last day, would I be happy with what I contributed to the world? And am I happy with who I am?"

The answer was a big fat NO. I, like so many, got wrapped up into what my life should be versus what I needed, wanted, and deserved. The work was difficult at times because staring our beliefs in the face, whether they are associated with other people, or recognizing how much we have contributed to our own misfortunes, can be devastatingly difficult. The way I see it, is that regardless of this pain, the sooner we can change this for ourselves, the sooner we can live happier more quality lives. Hopefully while preventing even more physical and emotional congestion.

With having always been interested in health and fitness, this opportunity for growth allowed me to step into a role that I never believed I was capable of. Sometimes we must knock down the building, repair the foundation, and reconstruct to really find the stability and balance. My eyes were opened to what it is like for so many people struggling daily with the symptoms I experienced. I believe my divine guidance only revealed to me what was happening in my body piece by piece over these past two years, so I could understand how often we look topically at things when many of us have a common root problem. Not just in the relationship we have with ourselves and how this attracts what we want in our life, but in movement, supplementation, and therapeutic ways to assist our everyday living in getting there.

Although all of this happened while I was going through my health coaching program, it lit a spark in me to further this life-changing opportunity even more. How might I be able to better embrace my own light and shine? I realized how much I stepped out of the way for others to feel center stage, as well as the negative beliefs I had for what "center stage" even meant. Now I see that I can positively share the stage with everyone and contribute in a way that makes me feel whole. "Can Amanda Gabbert really impact lives?" Yes inner dialogue, I can. So can you.

Additional education gave me a lot to go off of whether it be learning dozens of different dietary theories, self-care practices, and how everything about our being impacts health. I received my personal training certification as well, and although I wanted to think I already knew everything (hello ego), I learned so much more in how we view movement and what's really going to set us up for success. Whether we are prepping for a competition or looking to guarantee ease of movement in our Golden Girl years, there are many physical pieces we need to acknowledge outside of what's in the mirror.

The beautiful thing is on top of these foundations, my personal experience, hours of reading, researching and applying multiple theories to my own life, has shown me the numerous ways available to us for change and how to intuitively understand what works on an individual level. Along with clients, I have had many friends and family ask me questions regarding health concerns and it has been rewarding to share experiences and make referrals, while supporting their personal goals.

It took me a while to figure out what I wanted to focus on when it came to Health Coaching and Energy Healing. I knew I needed to decide on a niche in order to narrow down what a prospective client coming to me would want guidance in. The answer was right in front of me the whole time. Detox clears everything that might be congested- body, mind and soul.

YOUR WHY

What's going well in your life? What excites you about your day? What maybe isn't so great or exciting? Do you share any similar reflections on your life thus far and who you want to be? What do you believe you deserve? Too many of us assume that alternative health care is expensive, but although I spent a lot of money in my process, I came to see how we can work around this for all people, not just those who are in the middle to upper class. Outside of budget, we are also looking at the savings in all the prescription medications you might be able to toss down the line. This, plus ridding you of unhealthy habits will most likely save you money in the process. So, I ask you, what's more important? Quick fixes now and allowing toxins to build in your body, emotionally and physically, or working to add home therapies and holistic practitioners in your day before too much has accumulated? Some of us must have a tough experience to awaken the need for a detox, but others may see their future sooner, feeling there's no time but the present. Your threshold and my threshold are different, and we can all respect each other's knowing it will come up for us at the right time.

Letting go of all the familiarity we have grown with sucks. It's a death grip that allows some much-needed faith and hope to come in and the idea of trusting the abstract and unseen feels like assuming we can walk on air sometimes. We have come to thrive off instant gratification, working ourselves to death for a dollar, avoiding vulnerability out of fear of judgment and sizing ourselves up to the person next to us. What's so wrong with being different? Why should we not recognize what we can offer as an individual and allow others to recognize us for this, too? At the end of the day, the right people in our life will support us for who we are, while offering us equally emotional transactions in the ways we need. Know that this moment will come to you if it has not already, and experiences will become more fulfilling with change.

For those of us that feel like we've tried it all, or we are not getting the attention that we need, Health Coaching and Energy Healing could be an answer. With all that we have discussed thus far, we would include this in coaching and add small but sure changes to integrate into your day to day for long-term success. Energy Healing differs depending on who you go to, however my approach includes looking at the physical symptoms alongside the emotions you are dealing with, and then discovering how this is connected to your energetic body. Whether you are looking to upgrade your thoughts, connect spiritually or change your eating habits, Health Coaching and Energy Healing together or separately can allow you to experience support on all levels, customized to your goals. Some of us need a plan to either boost us or verify a good fit with a coach, while others know we need an overhaul and a lot of accountability. Just like the details, there's no one size fits all program either.

CONCLUSION

One of my favorite movies of all time is *Hope Floats*, and there's a line the grandmother says to her family, "My cup runneth over." I have always loved this quote and one of the reasons it stuck with me in the past is because I think I was curious as to what that felt like. I can say today that I completely understand it's meaning. After the fear of wondering what was happening to me and where it would lead, to finally being able to feel joyful and grateful for every moment, my cup is running over. Live your life full of love for yourself and for others, find what you are passionate about, and do what you want in life now, rather than convincing yourself it's better put off for later.

Break the walls down of your conditioned "box" and live everyday as if there's no tomorrow. Find a healthy balance to honor yourself and your loved ones daily, while fulfilling the other responsibilities that come with life. In my opinion, the purpose of this life is love and relationships, while connecting with your joy. We may need to have responsibilities to provide a way of living, but the emotional experiences are what will be in our memories. Allow yourself the honor of this and don't look back wishing you did things differently or told someone you loved them before it was too late. Although many of us have our differences and that can be easy to focus on, we have too many similarities to continue avoiding compassion and support for each other.

Detaching from control, fear and scarcity related to the ego and dropping down to your heart will allow you to not only begin to adapt to the above paragraphs, but it will create less resistance to what should flow to you. Be open to what comes into your path and know that you are always receiving what's highest and best for you soul's purpose. Whether this be considered a painful moment of growth, or winning the lottery, everything is happening for us to rise to the next level. By removing all unhealthy expectations and knowing this is true, going with the flow will become easy and effortless. The more we become this, the more we can not only accept where we are, but begin to manifest and co-create our life.

Accepting yourself at any given moment is more important than accepting situations. The relationship with ourselves is the only permanence we will experience. You bring uniqueness to the world and this action encourages us to see the same in others for their roles in our lives- whether it's a conversation at the store, a supportive mate, or the growth you might experience after a falling out with a friend. Some of us might be here to seek fame in the spotlight while others of us may have a pivotal force in someone's life. No matter how big or small you feel your role is, every and all actions spread like wildfire. Your uniqueness doesn't have to be measurable to spark change in the world and make an impact. We all do this every day, so acknowledge the beauty of this within yourself.

Life, like detoxing, is not always easy, but there is a benefit to every occurrence. Feel the emotions completely and learn to tap into yourself and your intuition. Integrate supportive, detoxifying habits physically and emotionally. The more we cleanse, the more we can pay attention to our inner voice, flourish in happiness, and trust the path we are on. Your body and your heart will guide you to a heaven on Earth, and health of every kind will follow.

THE DAMN DETOX

LET THAT SHIT GO:

_____

_____

_____

_____

_____

_____

_____

_____

_____

_____

_____

_____

_____

_____

_____

_____

_____

_____

THE DAMN DETOX

THE DAMN DETOX

AMANDA GABBERT

_____

_____

_____

_____

_____

_____

_____

_____

_____

_____

_____

_____

_____

_____

_____

_____

_____

_____

INDEX

1 Christian Nordqvist, Alan Carter, PharmD, "Cymbalta (Duloxetine): Uses and precautions," Medical News Today, (March 23, 2017): https://www.medicalnewstoday.com/articles/248214.php

2 Mahyar Etminan, PharmD MSc, Joseph A.C. Delaney, PhD, Brian Bressler, MD MSc, and James M. Brophy, MD PhD, "Oral contraceptives and the risk of gallbladder disease: a comparative safety study," Canadian Medical Association Journal 183, no. 8 (May 17, 2011): https://www.livescience.com/13769-gallbladder-risk-higher-birth-control.html

3 "Liver: Anatomy and Functions," John Hopkins Medicine: https://www.hopkinsmedicine.org/healthlibrary/conditions/liver_biliary_and_pancreatic_disorders/liver_anatomy_and_functions_85,P00676

4 University of Luxembourg, "Altered microbiome after caesarean section impacts baby's immune system," ScienceDaily, (November 30, 2018): www.sciencedaily.com/releases/2018/11/181130094328.htm

5 "Signs And Symptoms Of Copper Allergy And Toxicity," Tandurust, (March 4, 2011): https://www.tandurust.com/allergies/copper-allergy-toxicity-symptoms.html

6 "Mandatory Reporting Requirements: Manufacturers, Importers and Device User Facilities," U.S. Food and Drug Administration, (September 27, 2018): https://www.fda.gov/medicaldevices/deviceregulationandguidance/postmarketrequirements/reportingadverseevents/default.htm

7 "The Health Benefits of Gratitude: 6 Scientifically Proven Ways Being Grateful Rewires Your Brain + Body for Health," Mindvalley Academy: https://www.consciouslifestylemag.com/benefits-of-gratitude-research/

8 Simon N. Young, "How to Increase Serotonin in the Human Brain Without Drugs," Journal of Psychiatry & Neuroscience 32, no. 6 (November 2007): 394-399

9 Karl Smallwood, "Who Invented the Food Pyramid?" Today I Found Out, (September 27, 2013): http://www.todayifoundout.com/index.php/2013/09/invented-food-pyramid/

10 David S. Hilzenrath, "FDA Depends on Industry Funding; Money Comes with "Strings Attached"," POGO (Project On Government Oversight), (December 1, 2016): https://www.pogo.org/investigation/2016/12/fda-depends-on-industry-funding-money-comes-with-strings-attached/

11 Hassan Malekinejad, and Aysa Rezabakhsh, "Hormones in Dairy Foods and Their Impact on Public Health-A Narrative Review Article," Iranian Journal of Public Health 44, no. 6 (June 2015): 742-758

12 Johane van den Berg, "Why Eating Meat Injected With Antibiotics Is A Growing Health Risk," Longevity, (June 6, 2018): https://www.longevitylive.com/anti-aging-beauty/real-health-risks-antibiotics/

13 Yue, Wei et al. "Effects of estrogen on breast cancer development: Role of estrogen receptor independent mechanisms," International journal of cancer 127, no. 8 (2010): 1748-57

14 David Jockers DNM, DC, MS, "Do You Have A Copper and Zinc Imbalance?" DrJockers.com: https://drjockers.com/copper-zinc-imbalance/

15 Copper Toxicity and Hair Testing," Hair Tissue Mineral Analysis Experts: https://www.htmaexperts.com/copper-toxicity-and-hair-testing/

16 "NIH Human Microbiome Project defines normal bacterial makeup of the body," National Institutes of Health, (June 13, 2012): https://www.nih.gov/news-events/news-releases/nih-human-microbiome-project-defines-normal-bacterial-makeup-body

17 Bob Weinhold, "Epigenetics: The Science of Change," Environ Health Perspect 114, no. 3 (March 2006): https://www.ncbi.nlm.nih.gov/pmc/articles/PMC1392256/

18 Kaitlyn Berkheiser, "7 Health Benefits of Manuka Honey, Based on Science," Healthline, (March 29, 2018): https://www.healthline.com/nutrition/manuka-honey-uses-benefits

19 Blendtopia, "Natural Detoxifiers – Charcoal & Clay," Super-charged for Life, (March 3, 2017): https://superchargedforlife.com/2017/03/03/natural-detoxifiers-charcoal-clay/

20 Kristin Dahl, "THESE 10 COMMON HERBS ARE MORE POWERFUL THAN YOU THINK," The Chalkboard, (July 28, 2016): https://thechalkboardmag.com/everyday-herbs-to-detox-rejuvinate-heal

21 Leo Galland, MD, "What's Living in Your Digestive System," Huffington Post, (May 25, 2011): https://www.huffingtonpost.com/leo-galland-md/stomach-parasites_b_828565.html

22 Jay Davidson, D.C., PSc.D, "UNINVITED GUESTS: THE TRUTH ABOUT PARASITES," Dr. Jay Davidson, (November 9, 2016): https://drjaydavidson.com/uninvited-guests-the-truth-about-parasites/

23 Jon Barron, "Colon Cleanse: Death Begins in the Colon," The Baseline of Health Foundation, (December 1, 2014): https://jon-barron.org/article/death-begins-colon

24 Maria Transito Lopez Luengo, "6 Liver Cleansing Foods and Herbs for Cellular Rejuvenation and Detoxification," Conscious Lifestyle Magazine, (February 26, 2019): https://www.consciouslifestylemag.com/liver-cleansing-foods-herbs-detoxification/

25 Amy Meyers, MD, "6 Benefits of Infrared Sauna Therapy," Mind Body Green: https://www.mindbodygreen.com/0-12265/6-benefits-of-infrared-sauna-therapy.html

26 Joseph Mercola, DO, "Niacin, Exercise, and Sauna—A Simple and Effective Detox Program That Can Significantly Improve Your Health," Mercola, (May 4, 2014): https://articles.mercola.com/sites/articles/archive/2014/05/04/detoxification-program.aspx

27 Elizabeth Palermo, "What is Acupuncture?" Live Science, (June 21, 2017): https://www.livescience.com/29494-acupuncture.html

28 Bleakley, C. M., Bieuzen, F., Davison, G. W., & Costello, J. T., "Whole-body cryotherapy: empirical evidence and theoretical perspectives," Open access journal of sports medicine 5 (March 10, 2014): 25-36

29 Yvette Brazier, "What is hyperbaric oxygen therapy good for?" Medical News Today, (September 28, 2016): https://www.medicalnewstoday.com/articles/313155.php

30 Datis Kharrazian, PhD, DHSc, DC, MS, MMSc, FACN, "How and why to do a coffee enema," Dr. K News, (August 2, 2018): https://drknews.com/coffee-enema/

www.ingramcontent.com/pod-product-compliance
Lightning Source LLC
Chambersburg PA
CBHW051024030426
42336CB00015B/2714